Recent Results in Cancer Research 83

Fortschritte der Krebsforschung
Progrès dans les recherches sur le cancer

Colorectal Cancer

Edited by William Duncan

With 50 Figures and 51 Tables

Springer-Verlag
Berlin Heidelberg New York 1982

Professor William Duncan

Department of Radiation Oncology
Western General Hospital, Crewe Road,
Edinburgh EH4 2XU, United Kingdom

Sponsored by the Swiss League against Cancer

ISBN 3-540-11395-9 Springer-Verlag Berlin Heidelberg New York
ISBN 0-387-11395-9 Springer-Verlag New York Heidelberg Berlin

Library of Congress Cataloging in Publication Data. Main entry under title: Colorectal cancer. (Recent Results in cancer research; v. 83) Papers from the Third Symposium on Clinical Oncology, organized by the Royal College of Radiologists and held in London, February 1981. Bibliography: p. Includes index. 1. Colon (Anatomy)-Cancer-Congresses. 2. Rectum-Cancer-Congresses. I. Duncan, William, 1930–. II. Royal College of Radiologists (Great Britain). III. Symposium on Clinical Oncology (3rd: 1981: London, England). IV. Series. [DNLM: 1. Colonic neoplasms-Congresses. 2. Rectal neoplasms-Congresses. W1 RE106P v. 83/WI 520 C71931 1981] RC261.R35 vol. 83 [RC280.C6] 616.99'4s 82-3214 [616.99'4347] AACR2.

Printed in Germany

Typesetting and printing: Carl Ritter GmbH & Co. KG, Wiesbaden
Binding: J. Schäffer OHG, Grünstadt

2125/3140–543210

Preface

Colorectal cancer was the subject of the Third Symposium on Clinical Oncology organized by the Royal College of Radiologists, London, in February 1981. This publication of collected papers is based on the presentations at that meeting.

The purpose of these symposia is to encourage a multidisciplinary approach to our understanding and management of cancer. They bring together not only clinicians of different specialities, but also non-clinical scientists who also have made a significant contribution both to basic knowledge and to applications of direct clinical relevance. It is hoped that symposia of this kind will be a stimulus to increasing collaborative research.

Colorectal cancer is now one of the most important causes of cancer deaths. The incidence of the disease varies greatly throughout the world but is particularly common in North America, Canada, and Western Europe. The aetiology of colorectal cancer is reviewed and a clear description is given of the factors associated with its high incidence in affluent Western societies. There is still no evidence of a direct association between dietary constituents and colorectal cancer, and so changes in our dietary habits that might help to reduce the incidence of this disease cannot be advised. While research in this important field continues, improvements must be sought in techniques of early diagnosis, assessment and management. It is particularly in the assessment and management of patients with cancer that the advantages of a multidisciplinary approach are generally recognized. In the field of colorectal cancer much remains to be done to confirm the benefits that are claimed to be associated with many new programmes of combined management. The results of surgical techniques have shown a small but appreciable improvement over the last 25 years. Further improvements in survival rates will be the results of more rational selection of patients with potentially curable cancer for specific regimens of combined management. Experience has shown that substantial progress can be achieved only by the scientific evaluation of carefully designed, strictly conducted, randomly controlled trials. It seems that increasing numbers of surgeons throughout the world are prepared to subject their results to peer review and audit, and to accept the demanding discipline of multidisciplinary controlled trials. Such collaboration must lead to steady improvements in the definitive management of patients with colorectal cancer. It is hoped that this publication may encourage greater participation in these clinical studies.

I have to express my thanks to those who presented papers at the Symposium, all acknowledged experts in their fields, and to their colleagues who contributed to the published papers in this volume. I would also thank Mr Michael Jackson of Springer-Verlag for his advice and patient co-operation, and Ms Dodsworth and other members of the editorial staff who have helped in the prompt production of these proceedings.

My thanks also go to Mr A.J. Cowles, General Secretary of the Royal College of Radiologists, and his staff, who helped in the excellent organization of the meeting in London.

And finally, the able assistance of my secretary, Mrs Joyce Young, has to be acknowledged, who once again undertook much of the work of organization of the Symposium and of completing the manuscripts for publication.

Royal College of Radiologists, London William Duncan

Contents

P. Fraser and A. M. Adelstein:
Recent Trends 1

L.J. Kinlen:
Aetiology 11

R.S. Camplejohn:
Cell Kinetics 21

P. Earnshaw, A. Busuttil, and A. Ferguson:
Relevance of Colonic Mucosal Inflammation to Aetiology 31

H.J.R. Bussey:
Genetic Factors 45

I.C. Talbot:
Pathology and Natural History 59

E.H. Cooper and J. O'Quigley:
Biochemical Markers 67

D.J. Nolan:
Radiological Assessment 77

J.D. Hardcastle and K.D. Vellacott:
Early Diagnosis and Detection 86

R.J. Nicholls:
Surgery 101

S.J. Arnott:
Radiotherapy 113

J.M.A. Whitehouse:
Chemotherapy 126

W. Duncan:
Prospects in Management 135

Subject Index 150

List of Contributors

A. M. Adelstein
Medical Statistics Division, Office of Population Censuses and Surveys, London, United Kingdom

S. J. Arnott
Department of Clinical Oncology, University of Edinburgh, Edinburgh, United Kingdom

H. J. R. Bussey
Consulting Research Fellow, St Mark's Hospital, London, United Kingdom

A. Busuttil
Department of Pathology, Western General Hospital, Edinburgh, United Kingdom

R. S. Camplejohn
Richard Dimbleby Department of Cancer Research, St. Thomas's Hospital Medical School, London, United Kingdom

E. H. Cooper
Unit for Cancer Research, University of Leeds, Leeds, United Kingdom

W. Duncan
Department of Clinical Oncology, University of Edinburgh, Edinburgh, United Kingdom

P. Earnshaw
University of Edinburgh Gastro-Intestinal Unit, Western General Hospital, Edinburgh, United Kingdom

A. Ferguson
University of Edinburgh Gastro-Intestinal Unit, Western General Hospital, Edinburgh, United Kingdom

P. Fraser
Epidemiological Monitoring Unit, London School of Hygiene and Tropical Medicine, London, United Kingdom

J. D. Hardcastle
Department of Surgery, University of Nottingham,
Nottingham, United Kingdom

L. J. Kinlen
Cancer Research Campaign, Radcliffe Infirmary,
Oxford, United Kingdom

R. J. Nicholls
St Mark's Hospital and St Bartholomew's Hospital,
London, United Kingdom

D. J. Nolan
Department of Diagnostic Radiology, John Radcliffe Hospital,
Oxford, United Kingdom

J. O'Quigley
Unit for Cancer Research, University of Leeds,
Leeds, United Kingdom

I. C. Talbot
Department of Pathology, University of Leicester,
Leicester, United Kingdom

K. D. Vellacott
Department of Surgery, University of Nottingham,
Nottingham, United Kingdom

J. M. A. Whitehouse
CRC Medical Oncology Unit, University of Southampton,
Southampton, United Kingdom

Recent Trends

P. Fraser and A. M. Adelstein

Epidemiological Monitoring Unit, Department of Medical Statistics and Epidemiology, School of Hygiene and Tropical Medicine, London WC1E 7HT, United Kingdom

Incidence

Geographical Variation

For some years the international scientific community has been engaged in filling some of the major gaps in our knowledge of the world distribution of cancer. This effort was coordinated originally by the International Union Against Cancer and recently by the International Agency for Research on Cancer. Collaboration between these organizations and a network of cancer registries throughout the world has led to a

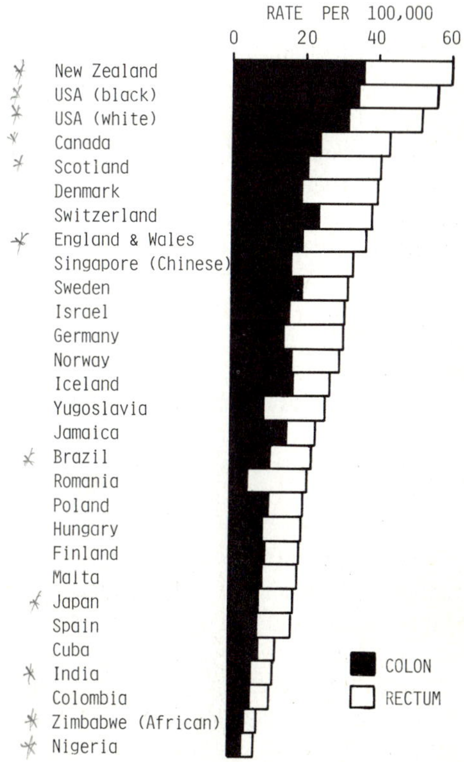

Fig. 1. Incidence of colorectal cancer: age-standardized rates per 100,000 males aged 35–64 in 1968–1972

Recent Results in Cancer Research. Vol. 83

series of publications entitled *Cancer Incidence in Five Continents*. The third and most recent volume (International Agency for Research on Cancer 1976) contains information on cancer incidence in 28 countries covering the time period 1968–1972. Hardly any investigator making inter-population comparisons in cancer epidemiology in recent times fails to make use of this valuable source of information. It has been used here to demonstrate the geographical variation in the incidence of colorectal cancer (Fig. 1).

The highest incidence is reported by cancer registries in New Zealand, the United States, Canada, and Scotland, while rates are generally low in Africa, Asia, and South America. The European registries assume an intermediate position, though Western Europe and Scandinavia generally have higher rates than Eastern Europe and the Balkans. Although it is predominantly a disease of developed countries Japan presents an exception, being a highly industrialized nation with a low incidence of large-bowel cancer.

In Fig. 1 the male incidence rates for colorectal cancer have been arranged in descending order of magnitude. A representative figure has been calculated when a country has data from more than one registry. The rates have been adjusted to permit a valid comparison between populations with differing age structures. They have also been restricted to a comparison of incidence at ages 35–64, to remove the distortion in rates which may occur with under-reporting in the older age groups, the degree of which may vary between countries.

The incidence rates show a nine-fold difference between Nigeria, represented by data from Ibadan, and New Zealand, where a national registration scheme covers the whole country. The very high rates in New Zealand are not shared by the small Maori population. The contrast between the American negroes, who now have an incidence of large-bowel cancer comparable to that of caucasians, and the low rates in West Africa, from where many of their forefathers came some seven generations ago, emphasizes the importance of environmental factors in the aetiology of the disease (Burkitt 1971).

For neoplasms of the caecum to the descending colon and of the lower rectum, a fair degree of reliability can be placed on the localization as stated by the radiologist or surgeon. By contrast, it may be very difficult to decide whether a neoplasm has arisen in the lower part of the sigmoid colon or at the rectosigmoid junction. A sigmoid lesion is classified according to the 8th revision of the International Classification of diseases (Word Health Organization 1967) with other colonic neoplasms as 153, whereas a tumour arising at the rectosigmoid junction is classified with the rest of the rectum as 154. Most registries follow the International Classification of Diseases and include the rectosigmoid junction as part of the rectum.

Rectosigmoid lesions may account for 15%–25% of rectal cancers in high-risk populations (Correa and Haenszel 1978), so it is apparent that diagnostic difficulties, local custom in coding practice, and some looseness of definition could give rise to spurious differences between populations when cancers of the colon and rectum are considered separately. However, in examining this problem in six selected registries recording tumours of the rectosigmoid junction separately, de Jong et al. (1972) showed that inclusion of cancers of the rectosigmoid with the colon, rather than with the rectum, resulted in only minor changes in the incidence rates. Classification artefacts are therefore an unlikely explanation of the pattern of incidence shown in Fig. 1 when the age-standardized rates for large bowel cancer are subdivided into those of the colon and those of the rectum including the rectosigmoid junction. There is a strong correlation in the incidence rates for these two conventional subdivisions of the large bowel, and, with a few obvious exceptions the colon-rectum ratios are close to unity. Lower ratios are seen in Romania and Yugoslavia due to a deficit of colon cancer, and the opposite extreme is represented by Jamaica, where colon cancer is twice as common as cancer of the rectum. Switzerland and countries with a very high incidence of large bowel cancer overall also have higher rates for colon cancer. The incidence of colon cancer closely parallels the prevalence of adenomatous polyps in all populations so far studied (Correa and Haenszel 1978). The collective evidence supports the view that an adenomatous polyp is a precursor of the majority of cases of colon cancer. Inherited disorders, such as familial polyposis coli, which if left untreated invariably results in cancer of the large bowel, and malignancy secondary to colonic inflammatory disease account for only a small fraction of cases.

Subsite Distribution

De Jong et al. (1972) made a detailed examination of the subsite distribution of large bowel cancer in 12 selected registries. They showed that although the incidence of large bowel cancer as a whole varied by a factor of up to 6 in their data, the pattern of cancers throughout the large bowel was similar in different populations. The pattern is illustrated in Fig. 2 with data from the South Metropolitan (now the South Thames) Cancer Registry (International Agency for Research on Cancer 1976). There is a gradual fall in incidence from the caecum and ascending colon (153.0) through the transverse colon (153.1) to the descending colon (153.2), with a sharp increase in incidence for the sigmoid colon (153.3). The rate for the rectum (154.1) is higher than that for the sigmoid, and the incidence of tumours of the rectosigmoid junction (154.0) and anal canal (154.2) is low. This subsite distribution is typical of large bowel cancer in areas of high and intermediate risk. A more uniform distribution of incidence by bowel segment is a feature of low-risk populations. When cancer registries are ranked in order of large bowel cancer incidence, there is a rise in sigmoid-caecum ratios as one progresses from low- to high-risk populations (Correa and Haenszel 1978).
Although the regular relationship between the subsite incidences in different countries suggests a basic aetiology common to all subsite cancers, there are instances where a selective increase at one subsite argues for a site-specific carcinogen. For example,

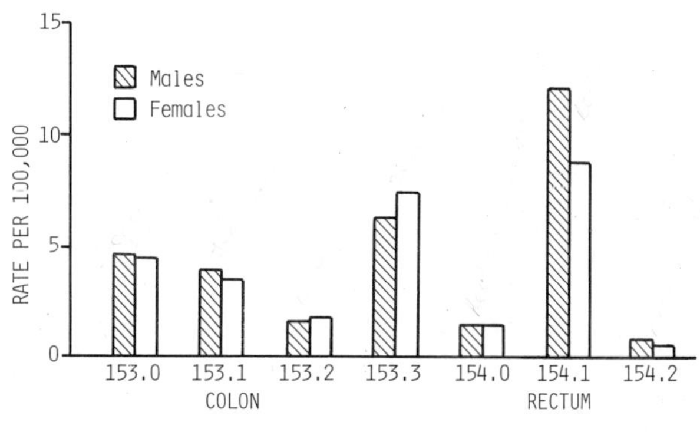

Fig. 2. Incidence of colorectal cancer by subsite from SMCR: age-standardized rates per 100,000 population aged 35–64 in 1967–1971

Denmark has a strikingly high incidence of cancer of the lower rectum despite intermediate rates for all other subsites (de Jong et al. 1972), and attention has been drawn to the relative increase in sigmoid cancer risk in Japanese migrants to Hawaii (Haenszel and Correa 1971). These segment-specific differences raise the interesting question as to whether large-bowel cancer represents a single disease or several diseases with different causes.

Sex Differences

Female incidence rates exhibit a similar ranking but a lower incidence of large bowel cancer overall, because rectal cancer is generally less common than in males. This is demonstrated in the male-female ratios in Fig. 3; in Fig. 3b few ratios are less than unity and male rates are on average 25% higher. Male dominance is also observed in colon cancer (Fig. 3a), though male-female ratios below unity are seen more frequently. Scotland, with a ratio of 0.74, shows the largest female excess.

Mortality

International Time Trends

Although 28 countries are now covered by cancer registries providing reliable data on incidence, an even larger number of countries compile mortality statistics for the major cancer sites. The World Health Organization has made these data readily available through the provision of computer tapes containing cancer mortality statistics for 33 countries since 1955. Although differences in treatment facilities and death

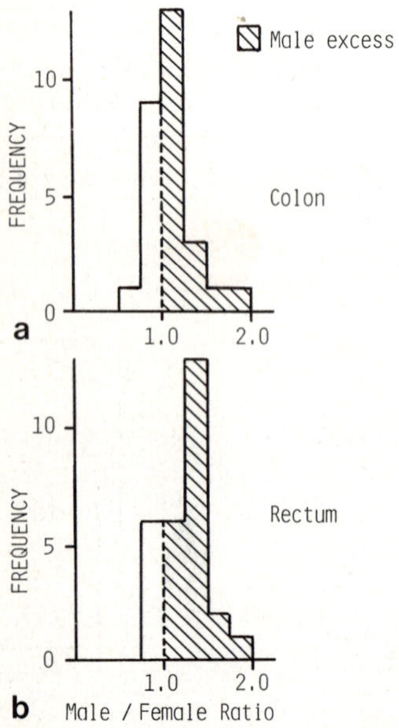

Fig. 3. Sex differences in cancer of the colon (**a**) and rectum (**b**)

certification practices will contribute to inter-country differences in mortality, the geographical distribution of mortality from colorectal cancer is consistent with the pattern of incidence (Correa and Haenszel 1978). These data from the World Health Organization enable us to examine time trends in mortality from large-bowel cancer in different countries over several decades. Selected examples are given in Table 1, the population of England and Wales in 1971 being used as the standard calculation of the age-standardized death rates.

A number of quite dissimilar international trends in mortality from colon cancer have been observed. Death rates in England and Wales are lower now in both sexes than they were 25 years ago. In Scotland death rates have also fallen, although the decrease has been relatively slow in recent years. With the exception of cancers of the lung and bronchus, colon cancer still causes more deaths in Scotland than any other cancer (Calman and Kemp 1976). By contrast, mortality in both sexes has increased in several European countries, the trends in Belgium and Czechoslovakia providing examples. Mortality has increased markedly in Israel and the Far East, particularly in Japan.

In many countries, including England and Wales, there has been a downward trend in mortality from cancer of the rectum. Scotland, however, has seen very little overall change, a fall in both male and female rates up to 74 years being compensated to a large extent by a rise in the older age group (Calman and Kemp 1976). Denmark had for many years held the leading place in mortality from cancer of the rectum in both sexes, but sharing in the decline, it has now been surpassed by Czechoslovakia, where mortality from rectal cancer is increasing. As a result of declining rates in the United States and increasing rates in Japan mortality from cancer of the rectum has become almost equal in these two countries, in sharp contrast with their very dissimilar levels of mortality from colon cancer (Logan 1976).

These diverse trends defy summary or easy explanation but must be the result of many factors acting in different directions and to varying degrees upon the different sexes and on different age groups and cohorts in the different countries.

Table 1. Mortality trends in selected countries: Age-standardised rates per 100,000 in 1955, 1965, and 1975

Country	Colon						Rectum					
	Male			Female			Male			Female		
	1955	1965	1975	1955	1965	1975	1955	1965	1975	1955	1965	1975
England and Wales	19.7	16.4	17.1	28.4	24.0	24.0	16.0	13.3	13.1	12.1	10.9	10.9
Scotland	29.0	22.0	21.6	39.2	30.9	29.4	15.7	11.9	13.1	9.8	11.1	9.7
Belgium	13.5	16.3	17.6	21.6	24.1	24.5	14.9	13.7	11.5	13.0	12.1	9.4
Czechoslovakia	8.6	10.3	14.5[a]	10.0	10.9	13.9[a]	11.2	13.2	16.8[a]	8.5	9.8	13.5[a]
Denmark	16.8	19.1	17.4	27.2	28.1	25.6	17.6	15.7	13.8	13.2	13.8	11.1
Israel	6.3	10.2	12.9[b]	7.4	15.1	17.6[b]	7.5	5.1	5.5	3.8	5.1	6.4
Japan	3.1	4.3	6.9	4.2	5.9	8.1	6.0	6.9	8.1	5.7	6.8	7.7

[a] 1974
[b] 1972

Mortality in England and Wales

Time Trends by Age and Sex. The standardized rates considered so far provide a convenient summary measure of the experience of a population as a whole. Figure 4 shows instead the trends in four 10-year age groups in male mortality from cancers of the colon and rectum in England and Wales during the last 50 years. In all but the oldest age group the death rates for both cancers were very similar 50 years ago. Mortality from both decreased appreciably after World War II but the decline has been more marked for rectal cancer. Now, roughly speaking, one person in five in England and Wales dies of cancer, and one in eight of these dies of large bowel cancer. Because of a slight increase in male mortality from colon cancer since the mid-1960s, apparent in all the age groups shown in Fig. 4, the colon-rectum ratios have increased in recent years (Officie of Population Censuses and Surveys 1978a).
Female age-specific death rates show a similar postwar decline in mortality from both cancers, but female mortality from colon cancer has not increased recently. Male mortality from colon cancer increases more steeply with age, so that whereas female rates are generally higher below the age of 65, male rates are higher in the older age groups. Female death rates for cancer of the rectum are lower than the corresponding male rates at all ages, and in all but the oldest age group female mortality has been declining steadily over the last 50 years.

Migrants. Migration from Scotland and Ireland and an influx of immigrants principally from Eastern Europe, the West Indies, and the Indian subcontinent have resulted in a substantial number of deaths in England and Wales among persons who were born elsewhere. The unshaded standardized mortality ratios (SMRs) shown in Fig. 5 compare the mortality from colon cancer among male immigrants with the mortality

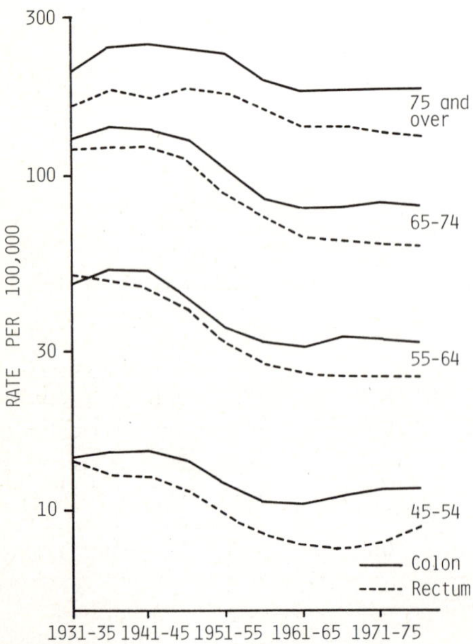

Fig. 4. Age distribution of male mortality from colorectal cancer in England and Wales in 1931–1978

experienced by the male population of England and Wales as a whole (Office of Population Censuses and Surveys, unpublished data). A ratio greater than 100 implies higher mortality among the immigrants and a ratio less than 100, lower mortality. The shaded SMRs similarly compare the mortality in the countries of origin with mortality in England and Wales. Mortality in the Indian subcontinent has been estimated from cancer registration data in Bombay because reliable mortality statistics are not available.

Studies of migrant populations, particularly in the United States and Australia, have shown that in general death rates from large-bowel cancer among immigrants tend towards those of the host population (Correa and Haenszel 1978). This trend is seen here for colon cancer, where mortality is tending to increase in male immigrants from lower-risk areas, such as India and Pakistan and Poland, and to decrease in Irish and American immigrants from higher-risk areas. The inference is that environmental factors, which may change on migration, are important in the causation of the disease. Mortality from colon cancer among female immigrants from low-risk areas shows a similar pattern, including an increase in mortality among West Indian women, although the data shown in Fig. 5 for West Indian males are not consistent with this hypothesis.

Regional Variation. In almost every country where regional studies have been carried out wide differences have been found in local levels of mortality. Regional differences between the standard regions of England and Wales have been summarized recently in *Area Mortality, 1969–1973* (Office of Population Censuses and Surveys 1981). In both sexes mortality from colon cancer is above average in the north-west region (male SMR 109, female SMR 107). In the West Midlands (SMR 103) and the north of England (SMR 107) only males show an excess. Mortality is particularly high in the large conurbations in these regions. Wales, outside the south-east, has higher mortality in both sexes (SMR 106) than eastern and southern England, where the SMRs range from 102 to 95.

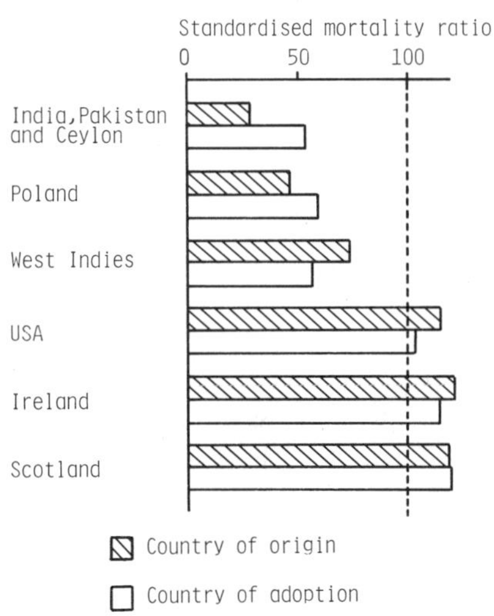

Fig. 5. Mortality from colon cancer among male immigrants in England and Wales in 1970–1972

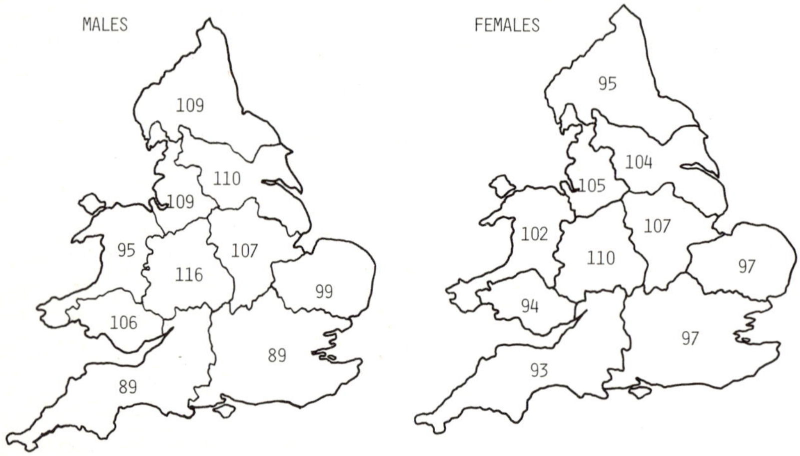

Fig. 6. Regional distribution of cancer of the rectum: standardized mortality ratios in 1969–1973

Cancer of the rectum shows greater regional variability in mortality than colon cancer (Fig. 6). Mortality is highest in the West Midlands in both sexes (male SMR 116, female SMR 110) and above average in north-west England (male SMR 109, female SMR 105) and the East Midlands (SMR in both sexes 107). Mortality is high only in males in Yorkshire and Humberside (SMR 110) and in the north (SMR 109). Dissimilar mortality patterns are also seen in the two sexes in Wales. Male mortality is above average in the south-east (SMR 106) but low in the rest of Wales (SMR 95), whereas the SMRs for females are 94 and 102, respectively. As with colon cancer, East Anglia and southern England experience a more favourable level of mortality, with SMRs of less than 100.

Mortality from colorectal cancer is higher in conurbations and densely populated urban areas than in smaller towns and rural districts, but the urban-rural differences are modest, rectal cancer again showing slightly greater variation with SMRs ranging from 107 to 94.

Social Class and Occupation. Male mortality from cancer of the rectum exhibits a social class gradient with higher mortality in the lower social classes, but male social class differences in colon cancer are small, mortality in social class V being only slightly higher (Fig. 7) (Office of Population Censuses and Surveys 1978b). Conventionally, the social class of married women is determined by their husbands' occupation. When classified in this way mortality from cancer of the rectum in married women shows a similar social class differential to that seen in men, with SMRs of 105 and above in the three manual classes. However, mortality from colon cancer is higher not only among married women in these three lower social classes (SMRs of 110 and above) but also in social class I (SMR 119).

Colorectal cancers are amongst the commonest tumours for which there is no clear evidence of a specific occupational factor. However, the *1970–1972 Decennial*

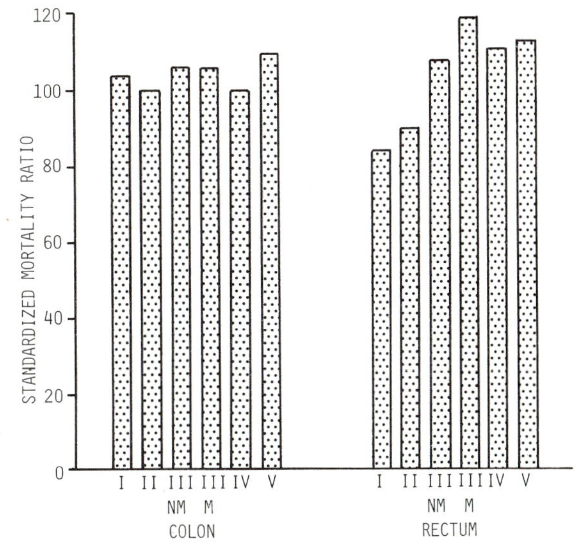

Fig. 7. Male mortality from colorectal cancer by site and social class at ages 15–64 in 1970–1972

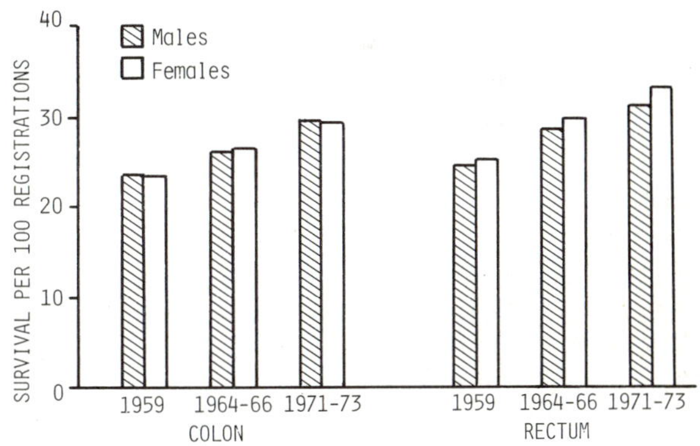

Fig. 8. Five-year relative survival (%) by sex and site of patients of colorectal cancer registered in 1959, 1964–1966, and 1971–1973

Supplement on Occupational Mortality (Office of Population Censuses and Surveys 1978b) reported high mortality rates for colon cancer in farm employers and managers (SMR 150) and for agricultural workers (SMR 136) but low rates for farmers working on their own account (SMR 69). Slightly higher mortality from rectal cancer was observed among engineering and allied trades workers (SMR 118).

Survival Data

Advances in treatment since World War II have improved the prospects for survival in patients with colorectal cancer. This is reflected in the steep decline in mortality in the post-war years when, for example, under antibiotic cover patients were able to withstand major surgery. Recent cancer registration statistics for England and Wales in 1971–1973 suggest that the prognosis for patients with colorectal cancer is still slowly improving (Office of Population Censuses and Surveys 1980).

The 5-year survival of patients with colon cancer increased between 1959 and 1964–1966 and increased again between 1964–1966 and 1971–1973 (Fig. 8). Even so, only 30% of cases registered in the last period were still alive 5 years later. More complete follow-up since 1971, with the National Health Service Central Register, and exclusion of cases detected only at death, may also have contributed to the apparent improvement in prognosis for colon cancer recently.

The prognosis for rectal cancer has also improved since 1959, so that over 30% of cases registered in 1971–1973 survived 5 years. By contrast with colon cancer, where survival is similar in both sexes, male patients with rectal cancer seem to fare less well than females. The prognosis for both cancers worsens with advancing age.

Conclusion

Recent trends in vital statistics relating to colorectal cancer reveal geographic, ethnic, and regional differences in the distribution of these cancers. They show changes in mortality over time and after migration, a higher risk in urban populations and the lower social classes, and generally higher mortality among males. The low rates of survival serve to emphasize that while clinicians are striving towards earlier diagnosis and more effective treatment, clues to aetiology, which may lead to prevention, must be vigorously pursued.

References

Burkitt DP (1971) Epidemiology of cancer of the colon and rectum. Cancer 28: 3–13

Calman KC, Kemp IW (1976) Gastric and colonic cancer in Scotland. Health Bulletin 34: 347–354

Correa P, Haenszel W (1978) The epidemiology of large-bowel cancer. Adv Cancer Res 26: 1–141

De Jong UW, Day NE, Muir CS, Barclay THC, Bras G, Forster FH, Jussawalla DJ, Kurihara M, Linden G, Martinez I, Payne PM, Pedersen E, Ringertz N, Shanmugaratnam T (1972) The distribution of cancer within the large bowel. Int J Cancer 10: 463–477

Haenszel W, Correa P (1971) Cancer of the colon and rectum and adenomatous polyps. Cancer 28: 14–24

International Agency for Research on Cancer (1976) Cancer incidence in five continents, vol III. IARC, Lyons (Scientific publication no. 15)

Logan WPD (1976) Cancer of the alimentary tract: international mortality trends. WHO Chronicle 30: 413–419

Office of Population Censuses and Surveys (1978a) Trends in mortality 1951–1975. HMSO, London (Series DH1 no. 3)

Office of Population Censuses and Surveys (1978b) Occupational mortality 1970–1972. HMSO, London (Series DS no. 1)

Office of Population Censuses and Surveys (1980) Cancer statistics 1971–1973 (survival), HMSO, London (Series MB1 no. 3)

Office of Population Censuses and Surveys (1981) Area mortality 1969–1973. HMSO, London (Series DS no. 4)

World Health Organization (1967) International classification of diseases, 8th revision. WHO, Geneva

Aetiology

L. J. Kinlen

Cancer Research Campaign, Radcliffe Infirmary, Oxford OX2 6HE, United Kingdom

The descriptive epidemiology of colorectal cancer in England and Wales presented in some detail in Chapter 1 gives little clue to its aetiology. Its incidence shows that there are no marked differences according to social class or to region of the country, and no marked change over time. Few occupational associations have been reported apart from asbestos exposure, and this has not been a consistent observation. Moreover, the finding by Newhouse and Wagner (1969) that some peritoneal mesotheliomas in asbestos workers were misdiagnosed and described on death certificates as colon cancers raises further doubts about the association. Nevertheless, the marked international variation in incidence together with the much lower incidence among blacks in Africa than in those in the United States point to the importance of environmental factors in the causation of these cancers.

Genetic Factors

The most firmly established cause of colon cancer is genetic, namely the gene for polyposis coli. However, this is responsible for only a very small proportion of cases in the population, since only about 1 in 10,000 people are estimated to carry this gene. Several studies have observed an excess of colorectal cancer in the first-degree relatives of affected patients (see Table 1) which is apparently not explained by the inclusion of patients with familial polyposis coli.

Dietary Factors

Genetic factors, however, cannot explain the marked international variation in incidence shown by this neoplasm or why migrants from countries with a low

Table 1. Colorectal cancer in first-degree relatives of affected patients

Reference	Observed	Expected	O/E ratio
Woolf 1958	26	8.0	3.3
Macklin 1960	31	9.7	3.2
Lovett 1976	41	11.7	3.5
Bjelke 1980	23	13.7	1.7

Recent Results in Cancer Research, Vol. 83

incidence, such as the Japanese in the United States, show an increase in incidence reaching levels in the next generation similar to those recorded in natives of the host country (Smith 1956; Haenszel and Kurihara 1968). Diet is one aspect of the life-style of these Japanese immigrants in the USA that is particularly subject to change. Wynder and Shigematsu (1967) were perhaps the first to suggest that fat might be the relevant dietary constituent, for they were impressed by the much larger proportion of calories in the United States than in Japan that were derived from saturated fat. They also pointed out the close correlation that existed between the average intake of fat in different countries and the corresponding mortality from colon cancer, an observation that has been confirmed by other workers and shown also to apply to meat (Fig. 1; Armstrong and Doll 1975). Further support came from a case-control study in Japan, where more individuals with this cancer than controls were found to have adopted a Western diet (Wynder et al. 1969).

Bacterial Flora

In 1971 Hill et al. reported a striking relationship between certain bacteriological and chemical characteristics of faecal samples collected in different countries and the corresponding mortality rates for large-bowel cancer. Samples from countries with a high incidence of the disease had a higher frequency of anaerobic bacteria, particularly of the type described as nuclear dehydrogenating clostridia, which can degrade bile salts. In addition, stools from high-incidence countries had higher concentrations of neutral and acid sterols, derived from the breakdown of cholesterol and bile salts, respectively. In the light of work indicating that a high fat intake increases the faecal concentration of bile acids (Hill 1971), these findings appeared to indicate a mechanism for the relationship between colon cancer and fat (or meat) intake suggested by the international correlation studies. Populations with a high consumption of fat appeared to have an intestinal flora with a greater capacity for breaking down the more plentiful degradation products of bile salts into putatively carcinogenic elements. Subsequent reports that Californian Adventists who eat little or no meat had a low incidence of large-bowel cancer appeared to confirm the above relationship,

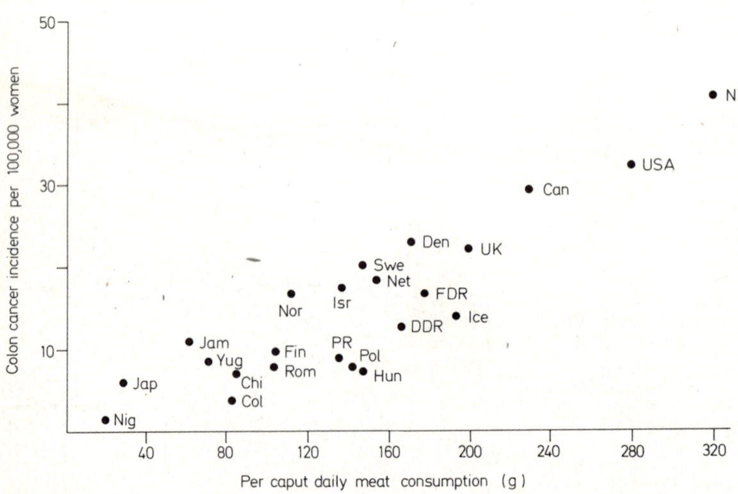

Fig. 1

Table 2. Case-control studies of dietary factors in colorectal cancer

Reference	Location	Numbers		Association	
		Patients	Controls	Positive	Negative
Stocks 1958	England and Wales	300	9,000	Beer	Vegetables
Higginson 1966	USA	340	1,020	–	–
Wynder and Shigematsu 1967	New York	791	409	Beer	–
Paymaster et al. 1968	Bombay	1,636	1,314	–	Vegetarian diet high in dairy products
Wynder et al. 1969	Japan	157	307	Fruit and milk	Rice
Haenzel et al. 1973	Hawaii	179	357	Meat, legumes, starches	–
Bjelke 1973	Norway	278	1,394	–	Vegetables, vit. A, coffee
Bjelke 1973	Minnesota, USA	373	1,657	Meat (rectum only)	Vegetables, fruit, coffee, crude fibre, vit. A and C
Phillips 1975	California, USA	41	123	Meat, fish, dairy products (except milk) in the past	–
Modan et al. 1975	Israel	275	550	–	Vegetables
Graham et al. 1978	New York	982	2,392	–	Vegetables

Table 3. Deaths from colorectal cancer in women in strict religious orders by meat and fat intake

Dietary group	Colon Ca		Rectum Ca		Colorectal Ca		O/E ration
	Observed	Expected	Observed	Expected	Observed	Expected	
Partially meat-abstaining	14	15.09	9	6.82	23	21.91	1.05
Meat-abstaining	17	17.28	6	8.05	23	25.33	0.91
Low fat	3	3.83	2	1.78	5	5.61	0.89
Medium fat	4	3.39	1	1.57	5	4.96	1.01
High fat	2	3.80	0	1.76	2	5.56	0.54
Not known	8	6.28	3	2.93	11	9.21	1.19

since meat is a major source of fat, though some specific effect of meat was also a possibility (Phillips 1975).

Fats

An obvious question raised by this hypothesis is whether individuals with large bowel cancer have a greater consumption of fat or meat than controls. Several studies have investigated this question, but on the whole with negative results (Table 2). This alone, however, did not necessarily weigh strongly against the supposed relationship. Dietary recall studies, it was argued, are relatively insensitive, and the fact that one of the few positive studies with regard to meat was conducted in Hawaii suggested that only such marked dietary heterogeneity as is present there might allow a relationship to be easily detected by the case-control approach.

Subsequent work, however, has not supported the seemingly simple relationship between colorectal cancer and fat. The International Agency for Research on Cancer (1977) studied the question in two areas of Scandinavia with contrasting incidences of large bowel cancer, namely in Copenhagen (high) and Kuopia in Finland (low). The Danes, however, did not have more nuclear dehydrogenating clostridia or more acid or neutral sterols in their stools, though they did have more anaerobic bacteria in general than the Finns. Moreover, bacteriological and chemical examination of stools from patients with colonic and rectal polyps (who are at increased risk of bowel cancer) and controls has not revealed the expected differences (Mastromarino et al. 1978; Finegold et al. 1975; Watne et al. 1976; Mudd et al. 1978, 1979; Murrey et al. 1980).

Meat

Kinlen (1980) investigated the mortality from colorectal and other cancers in members of certain enclosed religious orders who either abstained entirely from meat or only ate meat on less than half the days in the week. Table 3 shows that neither of these groups had an appreciably lower mortality from colorectal cancer than the general populations. It is, of course, possible to have an average intake of fat in the absence of meat, for example by having a high intake of dairy products. This does not explain the observations in the nuns, since an analysis in terms of fat intake revealed no differences between the low and high fat consumption categories (Table 3). Other evidence also weighs against the relationship. There has been an increased consumption of beef and fat in the United States since 1940, particularly of the former, besides appreciable geographic and socioeconomic differences in their consumption, but without corresponding changes or differences in mortality from colorectal cancer (Enstrom 1975). In addition Mormons, who have been reported to eat more meat than the average for the United States, have a low incidence of colon cancer (Table 4; Lyons and Sorenson 1978).

Vegetables

But though the case-control comparisons of diet reveal little difference with respect to meat, it is striking how many studies (see Table 2) have indicated a negative

Table 4. Standardised mortality ratios (SMRs) in certain religious groups in the United States

Religious group	Period	SMR	Reference
Californian Adventists	1958–1965	63	Phillips 1975
Utah County (85% Mormon)	1950–1969	63	Enstrom 1975
Utah active Mormon males	1970–1975	54	Enstrom 1977
Californian active Mormon males	1968–1975	64	Enstrom 1977

Table 5. Relative risk of colorectal cancer by intake of vegetables

Vegetable intake index	Retrospective		Prospective	
	No. of cases	Relative risk	No. of cases	Relative risk
Norway				
Low	101	1.00	47	1.00
High	177	0.76	21	1.10
USA				
Low	98	1.00	21	1.00
High	275	0.56	28	0.67

From Bjelke 1980

relationship between colorectal cancer and vegetable consumption. This has also appeared in a prospective study (Table 5). What constituent(s) of vegetables might exert this protective effect? One candidate is beta-carotene, the most important pro-vitamin A in man, which is present in large amounts in certain vegetables, such as carrots. Largely as a result of work by Bjelke (1973), there has been a growing interest in the possibility that a relative lack of vitamin A might be a factor encouraging the development of certain cancers even in countries where the classic picture of hypovitaminosis A is virtually unknown. This possibility is supported by laboratory work, and in several experimental models the yield of tumours in animals can be increased by reducing their intake of vitamin A.

But vegetables contain other potentially relevant substances, and in Britain approximately 40% of fibre consumption comes from vegetables. For some years, Burkitt (1971) has been stressing that the low fibre content of Western diets may be responsible for the higher incidence of colon cancer and other diseases in the west than in Africa. He has also suggested that the longer intestinal transit time and the lower stool weight associated with a low residue would tend to increase both the concentration of any faecal carcinogens and their period of contact with colonic mucosa. It was initially thought that this hypothesis was weakened by the fact that only a poor correlation exists when the average intake of crude fibre in different countries is compared with the corresponding colon cancer mortality rate (e.g. Armstrong and Doll 1975). However, crude fibre is far from equivalent to fibre in the sense used by Burkitt, namely the fraction of vegetable matter not digested by human enzymes. It is of some interest therefore that a significant negative correlation between colon cancer

Figure 13

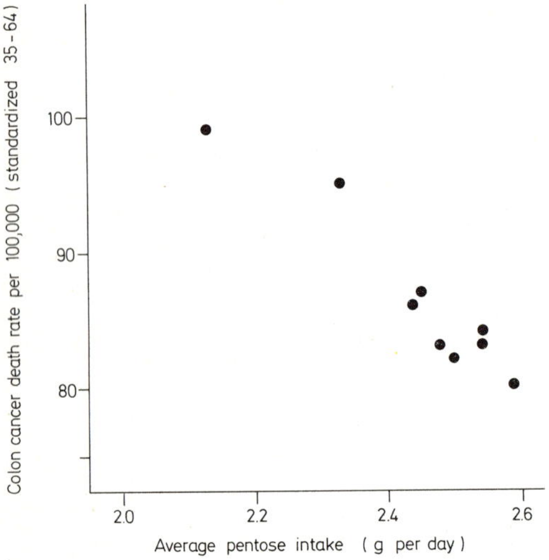

Fig. 2

Table 6. Relative risks of colorectal cancer by intake of carotene containing foods and by carotene intake

No. of high carotene foods eaten daily	Numbers of individuals		Relative risk
	Colorectal cancer	Controls	
0	67	100	1.34
1	66	126	1.05
2	47	94	1.00
3	36	75	0.96
4	23	62	0.74
5 +	13	47	0.55
Average carotene intake from the above foods			
< 0.5 mg/day	26	40	1.30
0.5 –	21	56	0.75
1.0 –	20	45	0.89
1.5 –	46	82	1.12
2.0 –	50	96	1.04
2.5 –	37	61	1.21
3.0 –	23	53	0.87
3.5 +	29	71	0.82

Data from Modan et al. 1975

in different regions of Britain and the average intake of the pentose fraction of total dietary fibre has recently been reported (Fig. 2), since this fraction appears to be of particular importance in increasing faecal bulk (Bingham et al. 1979).

Cabbages, turnips, and broccoli are examples of vegetables that contain appreciable amounts of indoles, which have been shown to reduce the yield of tumours in animals in certain experimental models, perhaps through their capacity to produce benzopyrene hydroxylase activity in the gut (Wattenberg 1971; Wattenberg and Loub

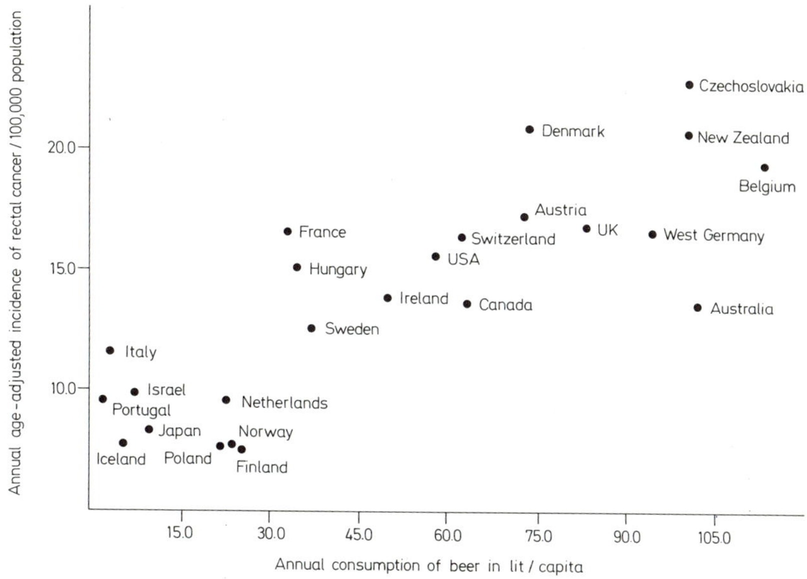

Fig. 3

1978). Relatively few studies have attempted to distinguish the possible effect of different vegetable constituents. Modan and his colleagues (1975), in a case-control study of colon cancer in Israel found a higher consumption of carotene-containing vegetables among controls than the cases, but when an adjustment was made for the actual carotene content the effect disappeared, suggesting that this had been due to a constituent other than carotene (Table 6).

Beer

A marked association between colorectal cancer and beer consumption emerged when Breslow and Enstrom (1974) correlated cancer mortality with the per capita consumption of cigarettes, spirits, wines, and beer in different states in the United States. The same relationship was again found in data from 24 other countries (Fig. 3). Enstrom (1977) followed-up this work by a more sensitive analysis in which he found that among cancers at eight major sites in males, rectum cancer showed the strongest correlation between *changes* in per capita beer consumption in different American states and subsequent changes in mortality. Furthermore, the male-to-female ratio of rectal cancer mortality correlated strongly with beer consumption in different American states. It is therefore interesting that Stocks (1958) found a significant relationship in the Liverpool area between intestinal cancer and beer drinking, while Bjelke found in a prospective study of 12,000 men that heavy beer drinkers developed colorectal cancer more often than those who drank less beer (cited in Enstrom 1977).

Two recent studies have investigated mortality from rectal cancer among brewery workers who are allowed a free quota of the brewery product. However, although a significant excess of deaths from rectal cancer was observed among Dublin workers (Dean et al. 1979) no such association was found in Copenhagen (Jensen 1979; Table 7). There are, of course, chemical and other differences between the stout

Table 7. Ratios of observed to expected deaths from colorectal cancer among brewery workers

Reference	Location	Period	Site of cancer		
			Colon	Rectum	Colorectum
Dean et al. 1979	Dublin	1954–1973	1.17 (32)	1.76 (32)	1.41 (64)
Jensen 1979	Copenhagen	1943–1973	1.08 (63)	1.14 (62)	1.11 (125)[a]

[a] Or 1.06 based on 140 cases

brewed in Dublin and the lagers brewed in Denmark, and it may also be relevant that both the national consumption of beer and rectal cancer mortality are higher in Denmark than in Ireland. It is clear that more work is needed to clarify this subject.

Non-Dietary Factors

Little evidence exists for non-dietary factors in the aetiology of colon cancer. Boyd and Doll (1954), however, found in a case control study of 614 patients with gastrointestinal cancer that twice as many affected patients as controls had used liquid paraffin regularly for over 5 years. It is relevant that in the period covered by the study liquid paraffin contained fluorescent substances that could have been carcinogenic.

Conclusions

There is sufficient evidence to indicate that diet influences the incidence of colorectal cancer, though not to incriminate any specific dietary constituent or its lack. The evidence appears to be more consistent for a protective effect of vegetables than for a harmful effect of fat or meat. Present knowledge hardly justifies strong advice about most dietary items of possible relevance, but it does provide further grounds for recommending a high content of vegetables in the diet.

References

Amstrong B, Doll R (1975) Environmental factors and cancer incidence and mortality in different countries, with special reference to dietary practices. Int J Cancer 15: 617–631

Bingham S, Williams DRH, Cole TJ, James WPT (1979) Dietary fibre and regional large-bowel cancer mortality in Britain. Br J Cancer 40: 456–463

Bjelke E (1973) Epidemiologic studies of cancer of the stomach, colon and rectum, vols 1–4. PhD thesis, University of Minnesota, Ann Arbor, Michigan, USA

Bjelke E (1980) Epidemiology of colorectal cancer with emphasis on diet. In: Davis W, Harrap KR, Stathopoulós F (eds) Human cancer. Its characterisation and treatment. Proceedings of the 8th International Symposium on the Biological Characterisation of Human Tumours,

Athens, May 1979. Excerpta Medica, Amsterdam Oxford Princetown, pp 158–174 (International congress series no. 484)
Boyd JT, Doll R (1954) Gastrointestinal cancer and the use of liquid paraffin. Br J Cancer 8: 231–237
Breslow NE, Enstrom JE (1974) Geographic correlation between cancer mortality rates and alcohol-tobacco consumption in the United States. J Natl Cancer Inst 53: 631–639
Burkitt DP (1971) Epidemiology of cancer of the colon and rectum. Cancer 28: 3–13
Dean G, MacLennon R, McLoughlin H, Shelley E (1979) Causes of death of blue-collar workers at a Dublin brewery, 1954–1973. Br J Cancer 40: 581–589
Enstrom JE (1975) Colorectal cancer and consumption of beef and fat. Br J Cancer 32: 432–439
Enstrom JE (1977) Colorectal cancer and beer drinking. Br J Cancer 35: 647–683
Finegold SM, Flora DJ, Atteberg JR, Sutter VL (1975) Fecal bacteriology of colonic polyp patients and control patients. Cancer Res 35: 3407–3417
Graham S, Dayal H, Swanson M, Mittelman A, Wilkinson G (1978) Diet in the epidemiology of cancer of the colon and rectum. J Natl Cancer Inst 61: 709–714
Haenszel W, Kurihara M (1968) Studies of Japanese migrants. I. Mortality from cancer and other diseases among Japanese in the United States. J Natl Cancer Inst 40: 43–68
Haenszel W, Berg JW, Segi M, Kurihara M, Locke FH (1973) Large bowel cancer in Hawaiian Japanese. J Natl Cancer Inst 51: 1765–1779
Higginson J (1966) Etiologic factors in gastrointestinal cancer in man. J Natl Cancer Inst 37: 527–345
Hill MJ (1971) The effect of some factors on the faecal concentration of acid steroids, neutral steroids and urobilins. J Pathol 104: 239–245
Hill MJ, Drasar BS, Ares VC, Crowther JS, Hawkesworth GM, Williams REO (1971) Bacteria and aetiology of cancer of the large bowel. Lancet 1: 95–100
International Agency for Research on Cancer, Intestinal Microecology Group (1977) Dietary fibre, transit time, faecal bacteria, steroids and colon cancer in two Scandinavian populations. (Report) Lancet 2: 207–211
Jensen OM (1979) Cancer morbidity and causes of death among Danish brewery workers. Int J Cancer 23: 454–463
Kinlen LJ (1980) Mortality in relation to abstinence from meat in certain orders of religious sisters in Britain. Cancer incidence in defined populations. Cold Spring Harbor Laboratory, Cold Spring Harbor (Banbury report no. 4)
Lovett E (1976) Family studies in cancer of the colon and rectum. Br J Surg 63: 13–18
Lyon JL, Sorenson AW (1978) Colon cancer in a low-risk population. Am J Clin Nutr 31: 5227–5230
Macklin M (1960) Inheritance of cancer of the stomach and large intestine in man. J Natl Cancer Inst 24: 551–571
Mastromarino AJ, Reddy BS, Wynder EL (1978) Fecal profiles of anaerobic microflora of large bowel cancer patients and patients with non-hereditary large bowel polyp. Cancer Res 35: 3407–3417
Modan B, Barell V, Lubin F, Modan M, Greenberg RA (1975) Low-fibre intake as an etiologic factor in cancer of the colon. J Natl Cancer Inst 55: 15–18
Mudd DG, McKelvey STD, Elmore DT (1978) Faecal bile acid concentrations in patients at increased risk of large bowel cancer. (Abstract) Br J Surg 65: 357
Mudd DG McKelvey STD, Norwood W, Elmore DT (1979) Carcinoma of the large bowel and faecal bile acids. (Abstract) Br J Surg 66: 355
Murrey WR, Blackwood A, Trotter JM, Calman KC, MacKay C (1980) Faecal bile acids and clostridia in the aetiology of colorectal cancer. Br J Cancer 41: 923–928
Newhouse ML, Wagner JC (1969) Validations of death certificate in asbestos workers. Br J Indust Med 26: 302–307
Paymaster JC, Sanghri LD, Gangadharan P (1968) Cancer in the gastrointestinal tract in Western India. Cancer 21: 279–288

Phillips RI (1975) Role of life style and dietary habits in risk of cancer among Seventh-Day Adventists. Cancer Res 35: 3513–3522
Smith RL (1956) Recorded and expected mortality among Japanese of the United States and Hawaii, with specific reference to cancer. J Natl Cancer Inst 17: 459–473
Staszewski J, Haenszel W (1968) Cancer mortality among the Polish-born in the United States. J Natl Cancer Inst 35: 291–297
Stocks P (1958) Cancer incidence in North Wales and Liverpool region in relation to habits and environment. British Empire Cancer Campaign, London (35th annual report, suppl 2: 2)
Watne AL, Lai HYL, Mance T, Core S (1976) Fecal steroids and bacterial flora in patients with polyposis coli. Am J Surg 131: 42–46
Wattenberg LW (1971) Studies of polycyclic hydrocarbon hydroxylases of the intestine possibly related to cancer. Cancer 28: 99–102
Wattenberg LW, Loub WD (1978) Inhibition of polycyclic aromatic hydrocarbon-induced neoplasia by naturally occuring indoles. Cancer Res 38: 1410–1413
Woolf CM (1958) A genetic study of carcinoma of the large intestine. Am J Hum Genet 10: 42–47
Wynder E, Shigematsu T (1967) Environmental factors of cases of the colon and rectum. Cancer 20: 1520–1561
Wynder E, Kajitani T, Ishikawa S, Dodo H, Takono A (1969) Environmental factors of cancer of the colon and rectum. II. Japanese epidemiological data. Cancer 23: 1210–1220

Cell Kinetics

R. S. Camplejohn

Richard Dimbleby Department of Cancer Research, St Thomas's Hospital Medical School, London SE1 7EH, United Kingdom

We know that tumours grow but our understanding of the dynamic changes which lead to this growth is incomplete, particularly in the case of human cancer. Precise and accurate data on human tumours are unfortunately hard to obtain due to the practical and ethical constraints existing in human cancer studies. In this review an attempt will be made to draw some general conclusions about the cell kinetics of colorectal cancer from information already available. In addition, some areas of current and possible future interest will be discussed.

Normal Mucosa

It would be useful as a first step to take a look at the proliferative unit of the normal large intestinal mucosa, which is illustrated in a very simplified form in Fig. 1. The proliferative cells are restricted to the lower two-thirds of the crypt. At the base of the crypts are to be found slowly dividing cells (Sunter et al. 1978; Bone and Camplejohn 1975), which it has been suggested constitute the stem cells of this tissue (Chang and Leblond 1971). The stem cells, though probably only a small percentage of all proliferative cells, are important not only for maintenance of the epithelium under normal conditions, but also for its capability to recover from injury. Stem cells have long-term proliferative capabilities and are able to repopulate crypts that have been damaged, for example by cytotoxic drugs or radiation. Some progeny of stem cell divisions retain these 'stem' capabilities and thus maintain the stem cell compartment while others move up the crypts, where they may undergo a restricted number of

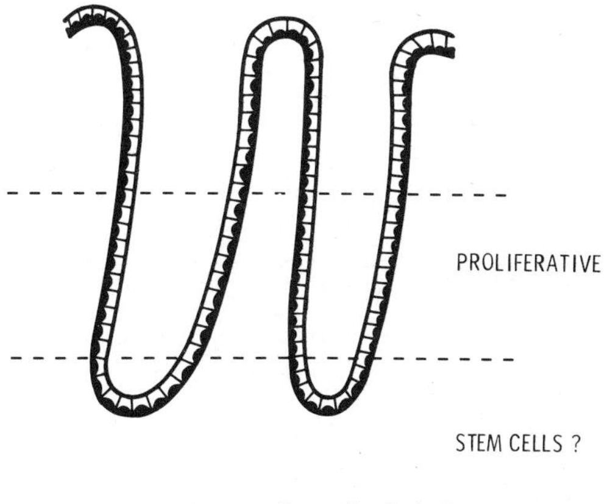

Fig. 1. A diagrammatic representation of the large-bowel epithelium indicating the location of proliferative cells

Recent Results in Cancer Research, Vol. 83

further divisions. In this way cell production is amplified to meet the needs of the tissue. The cells produced pass along a number of differentiation pathways to yield the various functional cell types normally found in the large intestinal mucosa (Chang and Leblond 1971). Functional cells eventually reach the mucosal surface from which they are lost. Obviously this brief description of the dynamics of the mucosa is highly simplified, but it is clear that this tissue exhibits an organized cell kinetic structure in which cell production, differentiation, and loss are balanced and controlled to meet the needs of the tissue.

Cell Cycle Events

It has been known since the early 1950s that proliferative cells pass through a number of distinguishable phases between one mitosis and the next. These phases constitute the cell cycle, which is illustrated in Fig. 2a. The period of DNA synthesis is commonly designated the S phase; the interval following mitosis and prior to DNA synthesis is called the G_1 phase; and the interval following S and leading into the next mitosis is called the G_2 phase. The time taken for a cell to pass around the cell cycle is called the cell cycle time (t_C). Cell population kinetics are, of course, more complex than depicted in Fig. 2a. In most real cell populations not all cells are in the cell cycle. The population is a mixture of proliferative and non-proliferative cells. This fact led to the concept of the *growth fraction* or proliferative index (I_P):

$$I_P = N_C/N \ .$$

N_C is the number of proliferative cells and N the total cell number. If some cells are not proliferating then the rate of cell production, otherwise known as the cell birth rate (k_B) will be slower than expected from the value of t_C. Thus the time taken for the cells to double in number will be longer than t_C and can be calculated from k_B, assuming no cell loss. This time period has been called the *potential doubling time* (t_P) and is also referred to as the apparent cell cycle time ($t_{C(a)}$).

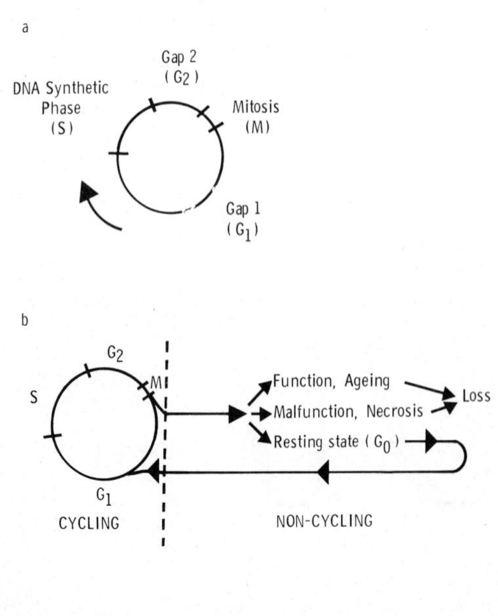

Fig. 2. The cell cycle (**a**) in its simplest form and (**b**) in a more complex form in which separation of cells into proliferative and non-proliferative subpopulations and the processes of differentiation and cell loss are illustrated

The actual increase in cell number, the growth rate (k_G), will depend upon the balance between the rate of cell production and cell loss (k_L):

$$k_G = k_B - k_L .$$

Cell loss is often expressed as a fraction of cell birth, and the *cell loss factor* is symbolized as ϕ (Steel 1968):

$$\phi = k_L/k_B = 1 - (t_{C(a)}/t_D) .$$

In this equation, t_D is the actual time taken for cell number to double. In a non-expanding steady-state system such as normal intestinal mucosa ϕ is, of course, unity. For a more detailed exposition of basic cell kinetics see Aherne et al. (1977a).

Application of Cell Kinetic Methods to Colorectal Cancer

Labelling Index

A great stimulus to cell kinetic investigations came in 1957 with the synthesis of tritiated thymidine (^{3}H-TdR), which is incorporated exclusively into DNA. Subsequently methods making use of this compound have been applied to the study of human tumours, including those of the colon and rectum. When ^{3}H-TdR is made available to proliferating cells, those which are in the S-phase incorporate it into DNA and thus become recognizable from then on. Exposure of a cell population to ^{3}H-TdR for a short period will enable the fraction of cells synthesising DNA to be determined. This fraction is called the labelling index (I_S):

$$I_S = N_S/N .$$

N_S is the number of cells in S and N, the total number of cells. This index is easy to measure in vivo in animals or, in the case of human studies, in vitro by incubation of tissue fragments or cell suspensions with ^{3}H-TdR.
Table 1 gives labelling data for colorectal cancer collected from the literature. Despite the small number of tumours assessed in most studies, there does seem to be considerable disagreement between the various authors. Apart from genuine

Table 1. Labelling index data for colorectal carcinoma

Reference	Number of tumours	Labelling index (%)	
		Mean	Range
Lieb and Lisco 1966	5	15.5	4.5–26.5
Wolberg and Ansfield 1971[a]	134	3.1	
Camplejohn 1974	4	20.5	8.1–32.0
Lesher et al. 1977	17	7.1	4.0–21.6
Bleiberg and Galand 1976	8	32.5	24.1–50.4
Bleiberg et al. 1977	1	35.1	

[a] 24-h labelling period

differences between the tumours studied there are a number of methodological reasons which might have contributed to this disagreement. However, labelling index data are beset by a more fundamental problem. Although I_S is often used as a guide to proliferative activity it is ambiguous, because the number of labelled cells depends (a) on the rate of entry of cells into S and (b) on how long they remain there. Thus, I_S gives no precise or detailed information about the cell kinetics of a cell population. More sophisticated methods in which ^{3}H-TdR is employed are available, however, and these will be discussed later.

Growth Curve and Doubling Time Data

The other early cell kinetic data on colorectal cancer came from growth rate studies. This information is derived from two sources. The first is primary tumours, the most detailed investigation being a double-contrast enema study by Welin et al. (1963) on 20 large bowel carcinomas. A mean doubling time (t_D) of 620 days with a very wide range

Table 2. Doubling time data for colorectal carcinoma

	Number of tumours	Mean t_D (days)
Primary tumours (Welin et al. 1963)	20	620 (range 138–1,155)
Lung metastases (Steel 1977)	56	95 (95% confidence limits 84–107)

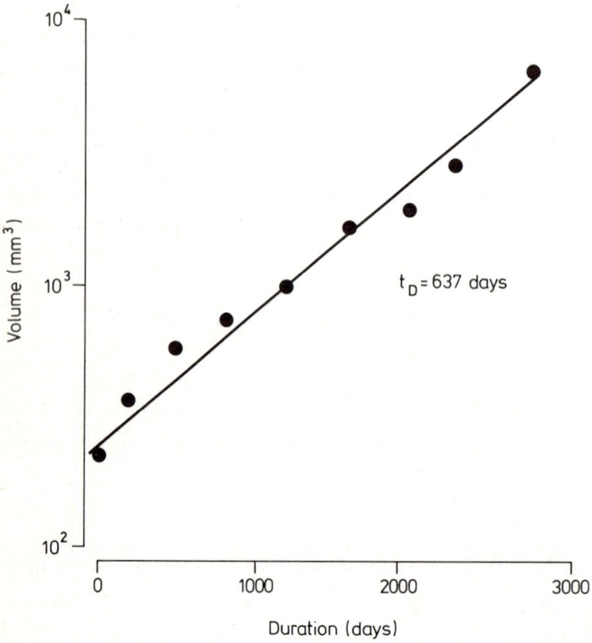

Fig. 3. A growth curve of a primary colonic carcinoma observed by means of a double-contrast barium enema technique. Data obtained from Spratt (1970)

was found (Table 2). The number of observations made on each tumour varied from 1 to 10 and was generally small. Figure 3 illustrates an example of an individual growth curve for a colonic adenocarcinoma in which measurements were made over a $7^1/_2$-year period. The data for this curve, which the authors concluded demonstrated exponential growth, were obtained from another publication by this group (Spratt 1970). The second source of growth rate data is from radiographic studies of metastases in the lung. Steel (1977) collected 56 cases from the literature, which had a mean doubling time of 95 days (Table 2). The data on primary tumours confirm the general slow growth of these tumours and also the wide variation between tumours.

The question of why growth is so slow will be addressed later. While it is necessary to keep in mind that the data for primary tumours and for metastases were from different groups of patients, it seems that the secondaries grew faster than the primaries.

Fraction Labelled Mitosis Technique

Under ideal conditions the fraction labelled mitosis (FLM) technique enables a detailed analysis of the cell kinetics of a cell population to be made. The cells to be studied are pulse-labelled and the fraction of mitoses labelled is determined in samples taken at frequent intervals thereafter. A theoretical FLM curve is shown in Fig. 4; identical peaks of labelled mitoses are generated each time the labelled cohort of cells passes through mitosis. Such ideal curves are never seen experimentally, because variations in the phase durations in real cell populations cause damping of the curves. Nevertheless, it is often possible with experimental systems to obtain two discernible waves of labelled mitoses, from which t_C, the phase durations, and I_P can be estimated. However, a typical FLM curve for an experimental tumour would involve (a) in vivo administration of ^{3}H-TdR and (b) 30 or more sequential tumour samples. Even if these requirements are met, which is not easy in clinical research due to practical and ethical constraints, large variations in phase durations may cause severe damping of the curve and prevent a second peak being obtained. Despite the difficulties involved, Lipkin et al. (1970) performed FLM experiments on both colorectal tumours and histologically normal mucosa from cancer patients. Two-peak curves were obtained for the mucosa but only a first wave of labelled mitoses was obtained for tumour. For this reason the estimate of t_C for the tumour can only be considered approximate. Lipkin et al. (1970) concluded from their results, only examples of which are given in this publication, that

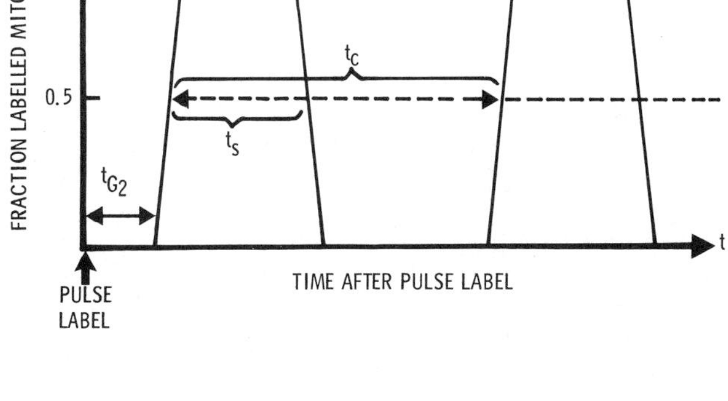

Fig. 4. Idealized FLM curve. Values for the cell cycle and phase durations are obtained as illustrated

tumour and mucosa had similar phase and cycle durations with t_C in the order of 24–48 h, t_S being 10–20 h and t_{G2} being > 8 h.

Stathmokinetic Technique

Rectal carcinoma and mucosa have also been studied by the metaphase-arrest or stathmokinetic method (Camplejohn et al. 1973). Stathmokinetic agents such as vincristine cause arrest and accumulation of proliferative cells in the metaphase stage of mitosis. The birth or cell production rate (k_B) is given by the rate of accumulation of arrested metaphases. Once again ethical constraints limited the number of biopsies performed for each patient, resulting in low precision of the estimates obtained. Patients were given vincristine IV following a control biopsy, and one or two post-vincristine biopsies were then obtained. Tumour samples were taken from 21 patients, from 11 of whom histologically normal mucosa was also obtained. The results shown in Fig. 5 demonstrate a higher mean rate of cell production in the mucosa than in the tumours. Mean values of $t_{C(a)}$ calculated from these data were 190 h for the tumour and 85 h for the normal mucosa.

Comparison of Growth Curve, FLM, and Stathmokinetic Results

Earlier we discussed the relationship of t_C, $t_{C(a)}$ and t_D to each other. This relationship is illustrated diagrammatically in Fig. 6. Comparison of the value for $t_{C(a)}$ from the stathmokinetic study (Camplejohn et al. 1973) with t_C from the FLM study (Lipkin et al. 1970) allows an estimate of I_P to be made. Further, the cell loss factor ϕ can be calculated from a comparison of $t_{C(a)}$ with t_D (Welin et al. 1963). The results of these calculations for both tumour and histologically normal mucosa are given in Table 3.3. It must be stressed that the values for I_P and ϕ given in Table 3 can be considered only as a rough guide for two reasons.

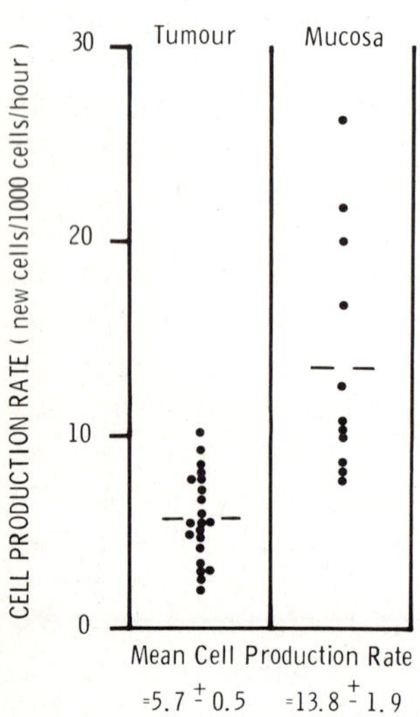

Fig. 5. Cell production rates for rectal carcinoma and histologically normal mucosa

t_C = cell cycle time

↑

only equal if growth fraction is unity

↓

$t_{C(a)}$ = apparent cell cycle time or potential doubling time

↑

only equal if no cell loss

↓

t_D = doubling time

Fig. 6. A scheme showing the relationships of the cell cycle time (t_C), the apparent cell cycle time, ($t_{C(a)}$) and the doubling time t_D

Table 3. Summary of cell kinetics for colorectal carcinoma and normal mucosa

	t_C[a] (h)	$t_{C(a)}$[b] (h)	t_D[c] (h)	I_P[a, b]	ϕ[b, c]
Tumour	24–48	190	15,000	0.13–0.25	0.98
Mucosa	24–48	85	–	0.28–0.56 0.56[d]	1.00

[a] Lipkin 1970
[b] Camplejohn et al. 1973
[c] Welin et al. 1963
[d] Bone and Camplejohn 1975

Firstly, the data from which they were calculated is of varying statistical reliability. Secondly, the experiments which yielded the data came from different groups of patients. Furthermore, these calculations tell us nothing about individual tumours and the differences between them. Nevertheless, if the general picture which emerges from Table 3 is correct a number of interesting points can be made. The cell production rate in the tumours is not higher than in the normal mucosa. Indeed it may be lower due to the larger number of non-proliferative cells present. Interestingly, Lesher et al. (1977) also demonstrated a high number of non-proliferative cells when they used an in vitro test for growth fraction. These authors reported a mean I_P of 0.30, with individual estimates ranging from 0.07 to 0.49. Another important point to be gleaned from Table 3 concerns the cell loss factor. Growth of these tumours is due to a small reduction in cell loss from the normal steady-state value of 1 to 0.98 (i.e., for each 100 cells formed by mitosis 98 are lost by death or other means). Growth is slow because the reduction in cell loss is small.

Clinically detectable tumours are already at an advanced stage along their growth curve; for this reason we have no direct information on the cell kinetic changes that occur during the early stages of tumour development in man. However, the data in Table 3 suggest that a higher proliferative rate than in the tissue of origin is not necessarily a fundamental property of tumours. It seems likely that the loss of the normal dynamic organization of a tissue and the resulting loss of balance between cell birth and cell loss may be more critical. In a mouse model of carcinogenesis Chang (1978) suggested that during transformation, stem cells with long-term proliferative capabilities at the base of the crypt failed to differentiate as they moved up the crypt. Such cells were then found higher up than normal in the crypt and tumours were seen to arise in the upper portions of the crypt. Thus in the very early stages of tumour development the normal pathways of differentiation were disturbed. Once this order is lost tumour growth does not require that cell production be higher than in the surrounding tissue, provided a small increment of tumour cells formed by mitosis is not lost.

Tumour Heterogeneity

Many studies with experimental tumour systems have demonstrated that individual tumours are heterogeneous. They may contain subpopulations of cells which vary in a wide range of properties such as sensitivity to drugs (Barranco et al. 1972; Hakansson and Tropé 1974; Heppner et al. 1978), metastatic potential (Fidler 1978), and cell kinetics (Gray and Pierce 1964; Hermens and Barendsen 1967). These papers are only a few of the many which might be quoted to demonstrate the wide range of variations seen within single tumours. Though work on human tumours is not so detailed, it is clear that human tumours are also heterogeneous. In relation to colorectal cancer specifically, Aherne et al. (1977b) demonstrated significant differences in mitotic activity from site to site within individual tumours. Further, Petersen et al. (1978), using the technique of flow cytometry, demonstrated the existence of subpopulations with different ploidy levels within some colorectal carcinomas.

Many attempts have been made to find correlations between kinetic data and prognosis, or response to therapy. Treatment schedules based on cell kinetic data have even been designed. Yet there is no convincing evidence that cell kinetics has resulted in improved patient survival or, indeed, been clinically useful at all. Two main reasons for this failure are apparent. The first of these is the poor quality of most kinetic data from human tumours and normal tissues. The second, and more fundamental, problem is the implicit assumption when labelling index, FLM, or other studies are performed that tumours are homogeneous. To quote single average values for tumours when they clearly consist of cells with widely different proliferation and other potentials is obviously of limited usefulness. The development of methods to enable recognition and measurement of the proliferative characteristics of the important cell subpopulations within tumours is very important. Specifically, the recognition of tumour stem cells is of prime concern. As discussed above, it is believed that stem cells are to be found in basal positions in the crypts of the normal intestinal epithelium. Even within the normal tissue it is not possible to demonstrate the location of these stem cells directly in situ, and in fact their location is still a matter of dispute. In tumours, which lack the high level of organization of normal tissues, it is impossible at present even to infer by indirect means which cells have 'stem' capabilities in situ. Such cells must exist to maintain tumour growth, to provide regrowth after unsuccessful radiotherapy or chemotherapy, and to give rise to metastases. Methods have been developed in which the clonogenic potential of tumour cells in a suspension produced by mechanical or enzymatic means from solid tumours is tested. Clonogenicity indicates the ability of a cell to undergo a certain arbitrary minimum number of divisions under artificial conditions. It is presumed that these cells, which are able to produce a relatively large clone under test conditions, may be the same as those with stem cell capacity in situ. This remains to be established, however.

Within experimental tumours the limited data available suggest that both the proportion of clonogenic cells and their proliferative characteristics may be quite different in different tumours (Steel 1977). Little is known about human tumours, although clones can be grown from some tumours in an in vitro soft agar culture method. Courtenay et al. (1978) obtained colonies from cell suspensions from two of six colorectal tumours.

Buick et al. (1980) failed to achieve any colony growth from four solid tumours but did obtain growth from malignant effusions of three patients with colorectal cancer. It has been claimed that such clonogenic tests may be useful both for screening new anticancer agents and for testing the sensitivity of individual tumours to chemotherapeutic agents (Salmon et al. 1978). However, the data presently available are not adequate for such claims to be confirmed. In all reported cases of colorectal cancer in which colonies were obtained, less than 1% of tumour cells gave rise to colonies. Much higher plating efficiencies have generally been achieved with experimental tumours. Whether this is due to suboptimal culture conditions for human tumour cells or whether it indicates a genuinely small fraction of stem cells in human cancers is not known. Despite the technical problems involved, the recognition of clonogenic cells and confirmation that they are related to stem cells in situ is a vital area of kinetic research. It is these cells, which are capable of unlimited proliferation, that are of importance to the clinical oncologist.

Conclusions

Colorectal carcinomas generally grow slowly. Cell production by mitosis in these tumours is not increased compared with that in histologically normal mucosa. Growth of these tumours is due to a small decrease in cell loss rather than an increased rate of cell proliferation. It is because the rate of cell loss is only slightly lower than the rate of cell production that the growth rate of these tumours is so slow.

Individual tumours contain a heterogeneous population of cells. The recognition of functionally important subpopulations of cells within tumours is an area of importance in current kinetic research. Of prime concern are cells with the capability of unlimited proliferation, which maintain tumour growth, cause regrowth after inadequate treatment, and give rise to metastases.

References

Aherne WA, Camplejohn RS, Wright NA (1977a) An introduction to cell population kinetics. Eward Arnold, London

Aherne WA, Camplejohn RS, Al-Wiswasy M, Ford D, Kellerer AM (1977b) Assessment of inherent fluctuations of mitotic and labelling indices of human tumours. Br J Cancer 36: 577–582

Barranco SC, Ho DHW, Drewinko B, Romsdahl MM, Humphrey RM (1972) Differential sensitivities of human melanoma cells grown in vitro to arabinosylcytosine. Cancer Res 32: 2733–2736

Bleiberg H, Galand P (1976) In vitro autoradiographic determination of cell kinetic parameters in adenocarcinomas and adjacent healthy mucosa of the human colon and rectum. Cancer Res 36: 325–328

Bleiberg H, Salhadin A, Galand P (1977) Cell cycle parameters in human colon. Cancer 39: 1190–1194
Bone G, Camplejohn RS (1975) Rectal carcinoma. A two-part study of tumour proliferation and host cellular immunity. Am J Proctol 26: 65–76
Buick RN, Fry SE, Salmon SE (1980) Application of in vitro soft agar techniques for growth of tumor cells to the study of colon cancer. Cancer 45: 1238–1242
Camplejohn RS (1974) Cell population kinetics of human tumours. PhD thesis, University of Newcastle-upon-Tyne
Camplejohn RS, Bone G, Aherne W (1973) Cell proliferation in rectal carcinoma and rectal mucosa. A stathmokinetic study. Eur J Cancer 9: 577–581
Chang WWL (1978) Histogenesis of symmetrical 1,2 dimethylhydrazine-induced neoplasms of the colon in the mouse. J Natl Cancer Inst 60: 1405–1418
Chang WWL, Leblond CP (1971) Renewal of the epithelium in the descending colon of the mouse. I. Presence of three cell populations: vacuolated-columnar, mucous and argentaffin. Am J Anat 131: 73–100
Courtenay VD, Selby PJ, Smith IE, Mills J, Peckham MJ (1978) Growth of human tumour cell colonies from biopsies using two soft-agar techniques. Br J Cancer 38: 77–81
Fidler IJ (1978) Tumor heterogeneity and the biology of cancer invasion and metastasis. Cancer Res 38: 2651–2660
Gray JM, Pierce GB (1964) Relationship between growth rate and differentiation of melanoma in vivo. J Natl Cancer Inst 32: 1201–1210
Hakanson L, Tropé C (1974) On the presence within tumours of clones that differ in sensitivity to cytostatic drugs. Acta Pathol Microbiol Scand [A] 82: 35–40
Heppner GH, Dexter DL, Denucci T, Miller FR, Calabresi P (1978) Heterogeneity in drug sensitivity among tumor cell subpopulations of a single mammary tumor. Cancer Res 38: 3758–3763
Hermens AF, Barendsen GW (1967) Cellular proliferation patterns in an experimental rhabdomyosarcoma in the rat. Eur J Cancer 3: 361–369
Lesher S, Schiffer LM, Phanse M (1977) Human colonic tumor cell kinetics. Cancer 40: 2706–2709
Lieb LM, Lisco H (1966) In vitro uptake of tritiated thymidine by carcinoma of the human colon. Cancer Res 26: 733–740
Lipkin M, Bell B, Stalder G, Troncale F (1970) The development of abnormalities of growth in colonic epithelial cells of man. In: Burdette W (ed) Carcinoma of the colon and antecedent epithelium. Thomas, Springfield, pp 213–221
Petersen SE, Bichel P, Lorentzen M (1978) Flow-cytometric demonstration of tumour-cell subpopulations with different DNA content in human colo-rectal carcinoma. Eur J Cancer 15: 383–386
Salmon SE, Hamburger AW, Soehnlen B, Durie BGM, Alberts DS, Moon TE (1978) Quantitation of differential sensitivity of human-tumor stem cells to anticancer drugs. N Engl J Med 298: 1321–1327
Spratt JS (1970) Gross rates of growth of colonic neoplasms and other variables affecting medical decisions and prognosis. In: Burdette W (ed) Carcinoma of the colon and antecedent epithelium. Thomas, Springfield, pp 222–229
Steel GG (1968) Cell loss from experimental tumours. Cell Tissue Kinet 1: 193–207
Steel GG (1977) Growth kinetics of tumours. Clarendon Press, Oxford
Sunter JP, Wright NA, Appleton DR (1978) Cell population kinetics in the epithelium of the colon of the male rat. Virchows Arch B [Cell Pathol] 26: 275–287
Welin S, Youker J, Spratt JS (1963) The rates and patterns of growth of 375 tumors of the large intestine and rectum observed serially by double contrast enema study (Malmö technique). Am J Roentgenol 90: 673–687
Wolberg WH, Ansfield FJ (1971) The relation of thymidine labeling index in human tumours in vitro to the effectiveness of 5-fluorouracil chemotherapy. Cancer Res 31: 448–450

Relevance of Colonic Mucosal Inflammation to Aetiology

P. Earnshaw, A. Busuttil, and A. Ferguson

Gastrointestinal Unit, University of Edinburgh, Department of Pathology,
Western General Hospital, Edinburgh EH4 2XU, United Kingdom

This paper is concerned with two aspects of intestinal inflammation and colorectal cancer. In the first part we review the clinical and epidemiological evidence that patients with chronic inflammatory disease of the intestines have an increased risk of the development of colorectal cancer. In the latter part, experimental aspects of intestinal immunological reactions and their relevance to colorectal malignancy are briefly discussed.

Colorectal Cancer Risk in Chronic Inflammatory Diseases of the Intestines

Ulcerative Colitis

Idiopathic ulcerative colitis is an inflammatory state, of unknown cause, generally confined to the mucosa of the colon and rectum. The extent of the disease varies considerably, almost always affecting the rectum, but with a variable proximal extent. Patients also vary considerably in their clinical course, some having chronic continuous disease while others experience infrequent exacerbations and return to normal health and normal rectal histopathology between attacks.

An increased risk of colorectal cancer in ulcerative colitis is well established. Tumours are distributed throughout the bowel, and have several unusual pathological features. They are often multiple and frequently are flat, with an ill-defined edge, infiltrating adjacent tissue – similar to scirrhous tumours of the stomach *(linitis plastica)*. They are frequently highly malignant, with early metastasis, and often have a 'mucoid' or 'colloid' appearance on histological examination. Prognosis tends to be poor, with an 18.6% five-year survival compared with over 50% in other carcinomas of the colon (Slaney 1971). Diagnosis may be difficult, for the symptoms, diarrhoea and rectal bleeding, mimic those of the underlying colitis.

The duration of colitis from the clinical onset of the first attack is an important risk factor in relation to development of malignancy. Results of several major series are summarized in Table 1, and the cumulative cancer risk over several decades approaches 40% (de Dombal et al. 1966; Devroede et al. 1971; Lennard-Jones et al. 1977; Greenstein et al. 1979). Adenocarcinoma has been reported as early as 8 years after the onset of colitis.

There may be geographical or ethnic differences, for recent reports from Israel, Czechoslovakia and Denmark show a lower incidence of malignancy in colitis than other series (Gilat et al. 1974; Nedbal and Marathka 1968; Bonnevie et al. 1974).

Recent Results in Cancer Research, Vol. 83

Table 1. Cancer risk in ulcerative colitis

Reference	Years since onset of symptoms	Patient years observed	Number of carcinomas	Risk per patient year
de Dombal et al. 1966	<10	282	1	
	10–19	101	2	
	⩾20	69	4	
Lennard-Jones et al. 1977	<10	578	0	
	10–19	392	2	
	⩾20	181	3	
Kewerter et al. 1978	<10	1,398	3	
	10–19	429	9	
	⩾20	73	2	
Above series combined (Butt et al. 1980)	<10	2,258	4	1 in 564
	10–19	922	13	1 in 71
	⩾20	323	9	1 in 36

Patients who have a total colitis, affecting the entire colon and rectum, appear to be at greatest risk, but there is also a substantial cancer risk in patients with left-sided disease. For example, in a retrospective study of 269 patients with ulcerative colitis admitted to hospital in New York (Greenstein et al. 1979) there were 26 cases of adenocarcinoma of the colon. Carcinoma was present in 13% of the patients with total colitis, as against 5% of those with left-sided disease. None of the patients in whom disease was confined to the sigmoid and rectum developed cancer in that series. The median duration from the onset of colitis to the diagnosis of cancer was 20 years for total colitis and 32 years for left-sided colitis.

Age at onset of disease is apparently also related to cancer risk, but this may be because the proportion of cases with a total colitis is greater in children. In the report from Greenstein's group (1979) there was no apparent relationship between cancer risk and age at onset, but in another series (Diamond et al. 1978) duration of symptoms before development of carcinoma was a mean of 16 years in patients whose colitis had developed before the age of 20, and a mean of 25 years in those patients who were over the age of 20 when colitis developed.

The presence of so-called epithelial dysplasia (Morson and Pang 1967) is probably the most important cancer-related factor in a patient with ulcerative colitis. This term implies both a structural and a cytological derangement of the glandular epithelium, with or without elevation of the mucosa and with varying degrees of severity. The epithelial cells are enlarged and there is loss of specialization, depletion of goblet cells, and altered mucus production. The nuclei are enlarged, variable in size and appearance, and hyperchromatic. Their mitotic activity is increased and there is crowding of cells and a tendency to stratification with loss of polarity. The cytoplasm is sparse and may become eosinophilic. The rectal and colonic glands become irregularly branched and can assume a tubulovillous pattern (Yardley and Keren 1974; Riddell and Morson 1979).

The presence of colonic epithelial dysplasia can only be used as a guideline in relation to cancer risk, for in 12% of carcinomas complicating chronic ulcerative colitis there was no dysplasia in previous biopsies or in the colectomy specimen (Evans and Pollock 1972; Dobbins 1977).

The dysplastic changes may be patchy and are not always present throughout the colon. Multiple bio[illegible] particularly those taken at colonoscopy, are of value in establishing th[illegible] or absence of epithelial dysplasia, however. Occasionally the pathologi[illegible]ficulty in differentiating mild dysplasia from reactive hyperplasia, and [illegible]ative absence of inflammation will favour dysplasia.

[illegible]nt lymphoma of the colorectum is also a complication of chronic ulcerative [illegible]tis, and like carcinoma, tends to appear in patients with extensive and long-standing disease. The lymphomas also tend to be multifocal. There are no histological features which direct attention to a prelymphomatous state. The ratio of lymphoma to carcinoma is approximately 1:10 (Renton and Blackshaw 1976).

Illustrative Case Report

A male patient recently seen in the Gastro-Intestinal Unit at the Western General Hospital illustrates many of the features described above. At the age of 11 he had a 3-month illness with diarrhoea and rectal bleeding, which was not investigated. At age

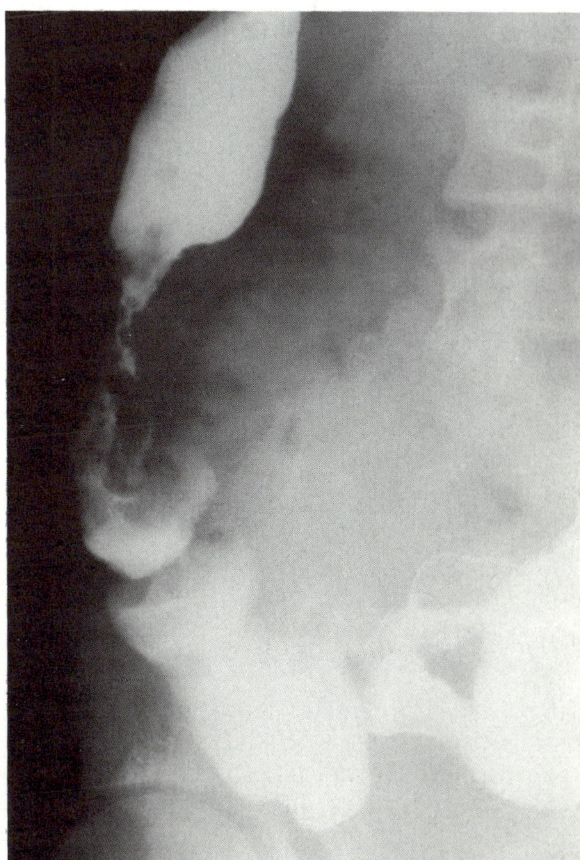

Fig. 1. Barium enema of a patient with total colitis showing stricture in ascending colon. Colonoscopy confirmed adenocarcinoma

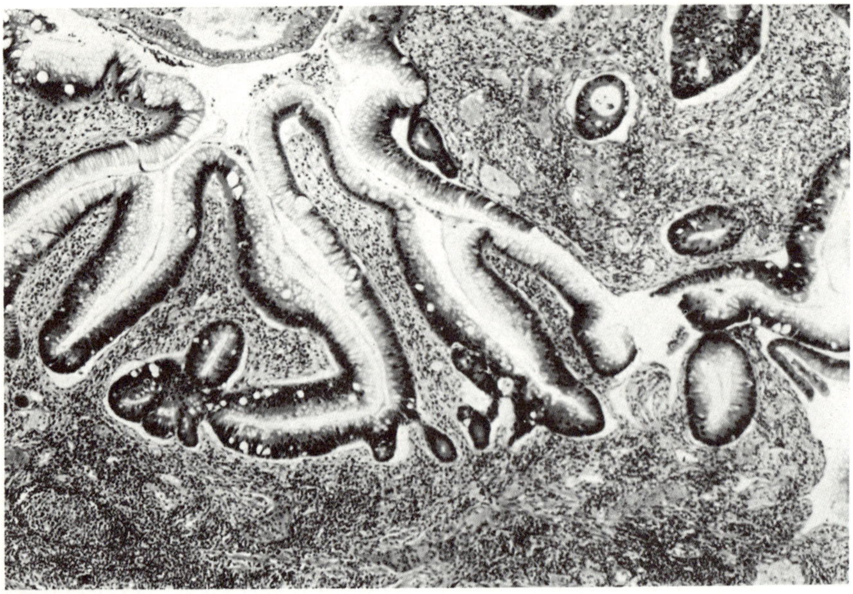

Fig. 2. Colonic biopsy. Chronic ulcerative colitis. There is irregular branching of the colonic glands. Loss of goblet cells, pseudo-stratification of cells, and nuclear pleomorphism are seen in the epithelial lining, particularly in the depths of the glands indicative of epithelial dysplasia. H and E; × 35

14 he presented with severe diarrhoea and was found to have confluent ulcerative colitis. Over the next 8 years he was treated with salazopyrin, corticosteroids and, for 2 years, azathioprine. He did not always comply fully with treatment and did not achieve complete clinical remission. In 1980, at a routine follow-up visit, the patient, then aged 22, reported no change in his recent symptoms (two or three stools daily with occasional rectal bleeding). The consultant physician carried out sigmoidoscopy and rectal biopsy and requested a barium enema. The indication for the radiograph was merely the passage of several years since the previous barium enema examination. Rectal biopsy showed mild dysplastic changes. The barium enema revealed a totally unexpected stricture in the ascending colon (Fig. 1) which was found at colonoscopy to be an adenocarcinoma. He underwent laparotomy with colectomy. In the colectomy specimen a second carcinoma was found in the transverse colon; histopathology showed extensive dysplastic changes in the mucosa in other parts of the colon (Figs. 2 and 3).

Crohn's Disease

This patchy, discontinuous transmural inflammatory disease may affect any part of the gastrointestinal tract. A relationship between Crohn's disease and colorectal cancer has been more difficult to establish than in idiopathic ulcerative colitis, for many patients with Crohn's disease are treated by resection of the diseased bowel. Furthermore, histopathological diagnosis of Crohn's disease may be made at laparotomy, and in some patients by endoscopic mucosal biopsy, but in many patients

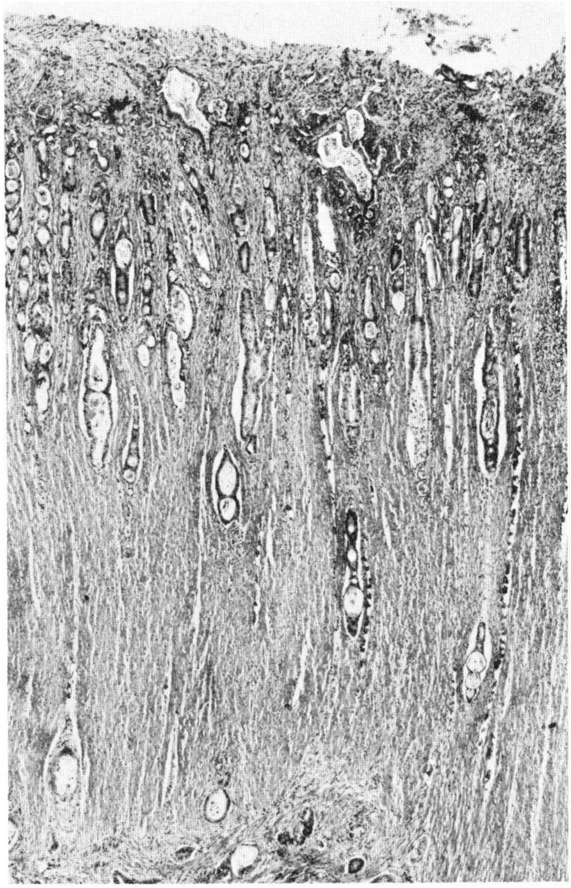

Fig. 3. Colonic resection. Ulcerated colonic adenocarcinoma of moderate differentiation arising in chronic ulcerative colitis. There are features of transmural spread. H and E; × 35

with clinically and radiologically diagnosed Crohn's disease no conclusive histopathological evidence is available.

Prior to 1970 there were a number of case reports in the literature which suggested an association between Crohn's disease and bowel cancer. In 1973 a large series of 449 patients with Crohn's disease was reported, among whom there were twelve cases of cancer, eight of these being of colorectal cancer (Weedon et al. 1973). This gave an incidence 20 times that expected, in relation to the age and sex distribution of the series. Two other reports confirmed a similar small but significant risk of cancer in Crohn's disease (Darke et al. 1973; Lightdale et al. 1975).

Although small-bowel carcinoma is a rare tumour, its incidence is also increased in Crohn's disease. Patients who have had surgery with bypass of affected bowel appear to be at special risk. In a personal series combined with a review of the literature, Greenstein et al. (1978) reported their experience of seven cases of carcinoma in excluded bowel, four in the small cases of carcinoma in excluded bowel, four in the small intestine and three in the large intestine. Of 46 Crohn's patients with carcinoma collected from the literature, tumour had occurred in bypass loops in 17 (37%). All of these patients with a malignancy had Crohn's disease of long duration before the development of cancer.

In a recent report of malignancy in Crohn's disease from Birmingham, an increased cancer risk was confirmed in a series of 513 patients, there being 31 malignancies in these patients. There was a significant excess of carcinoma in both the upper and the lower gastrointestinal tract. When analysed as patient-years at risk, with adjustment for the treatment of some patients by colectomy, the series as a whole contained nine patients with colorectal cancer, the expected number being 2.07; and in the 174 patients with 'extensive colonic involvement' the relative risk was substantially higher, with five tumours observed and only 0.21 expected (Gyde et al. 1980).

Coeliac Disease

Coeliac disease has a very wide range of clinical manifestations and is presently defined as a permanent intolerance of the small-bowel mucosa to gluten. The diagnosis is established by the appearances of jejunal biopsy. Although a frank colitis is rare, rectal biopsy does show chronic inflammation in some patients with untreated coeliac disease, and this reverts to normal after treatment with a gluten-free diet. It is likely that in the untreated patient some gluten passes unaltered along the gastrointestinal tract, even as far as the rectum, to precipitate the inflammatory changes there.

Studies of malignancy in coeliac disease have consistently showed an increased risk of malignant lymphoid neoplasms. Carcinomas of the gastrointestinal tract are also observed in patients with coeliac disease. In a series of 202 patients from Birmingham there were 14 gastrointestinal malignancies, including 5 colorectal cancers (Harris et al. 1967; Holmes et al. 1976).

A collaborative study, supported by the Medical Research Council, of malignancy in coeliac disease is at present under way in Britain. A preliminary analysis of the patients so far reported indicates that about half have 'malignant histiocytosis/lymphoma'; 25% have malignancies of the gastrointestinal tract, and 25%, other malignancies. Although there is a striking and significant number of patients with adenocarcinoma of the jejunum, few cases of colorectal carcinoma in coeliac disease have been reported to the register (C. Swinson and C. C. Booth, personal communication). If there is a significant excess of colorectal cancer in coeliac disease, the risk appears to be less than in the chronic inflammatory bowel diseases, ulcerative colitis and Crohn's disease.

Radiation-Induced Colitis

The evidence that chronic colonic damage associated with previous irradiation bears increased cancer risk is anecdotal. Black and Ackerman (1965) published a case report of cancer of the rectosigmoid 15 years after pelvic irradiation for endometrial adenocarcinoma, and collected five previous cases from the literature. Twenty-six patients with colorectal cancer following radiation for cancer of the cervix or uterus were reported by Castro et al. (1973). They found a relatively high proportion of mucoid carcinomas, and 58% of the patients had histological proof of radiation-related pathology in the bowel segments affected by carcinoma.

These reports give little information on radiation dosage, and further prospective studies are required. The highest risk appears to be in those patients who have chronic radiation-induced proctocolitis which is symptomatic over a long period of time.

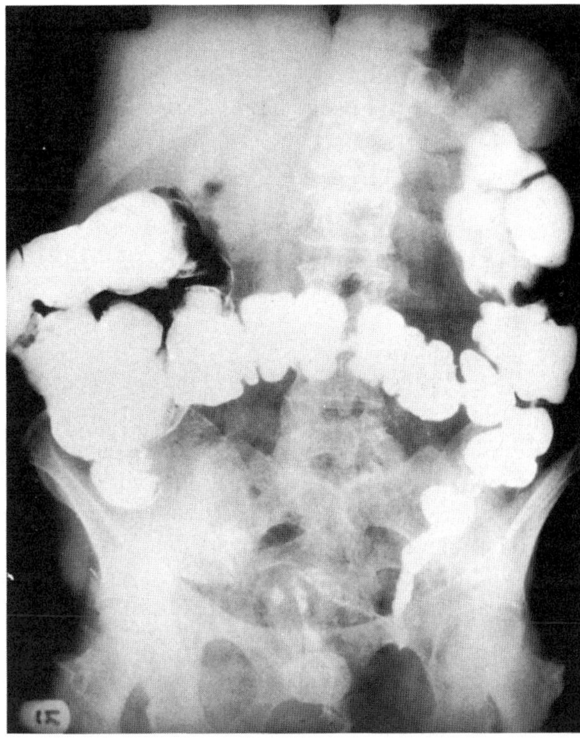

Fig. 4. Barium enema of a patient with a long stricturing adenocarcinoma complicating chronic irradiation-induced distal colitis

Figure 4 illustrates the barium enema of such a patient, who had a long stricturing adenocarcinoma complicating chronic irradiation-induced colitis.

Chronic Infectious Disease of the Colon

Amoebiasis. Although the clinical manifestations of amoebiasis may closely mimic idiopathic ulcerative colitis, an increased risk of colorectal cancer has not been reported in amoebiasis.

Schistosomiasis. The association between colorectal cancer and *Schistosoma japonicum* infection has been well documented by a report from Soochow (Ming-Chai et al. 1965). The authors had encountered 336 patients with colorectal cancer in a 15-year period, 90 of whom also had chronic schistosomiasis. The duration of symptomatic schistosomiasis varied from 5 to 20 years. Evidence that the malignancies occurring in patients with chronic schistosomiasis were different from those in the non-infected group was provided by comparison of the mean ages of the patients with schistosomiasis/cancer (36.9 years) and other cancer patients (46.7 years).
In the schistosomiasis/cancer patients, a substantial proportion of the tumours were multicentric carcinomas. Tumours in schistosoma-infected patients were typically distributed, with 66% being in the rectosigmoid region. This, of course, is also the maximal site of infection with the parasite. Pathological examination showed that the tumours were not related to the presence of ova in the vicinity, but appeared to arise in the areas of regeneration and repair of the mucosa, in polyps, and in ulcers.

Tuberculosis. Chronic tuberculous infection of the bowel may, perhaps, be associated with increased risk of malignancy. We have recently seen two patients, both female, in whom adenocarcinoma developed many years after surgery for tuberculous strictures. In one woman, surgery had been carried out when she was 7 years old, and a very large carcinoma involving the ileocolic anastomosis developed at age 51. The second patient had miliary tuberculosis as an infant and underwent surgery for tuberculous peritonitis at age 25. She required many operations and resections, and an intestinal bypass with chronic fistula formation. When she was 73 years old the discharge from a very long-standing fistula was found to contain adenocarcinoma cells.

Immunodeficiency

Primary immunodeficiency disease is frequently complicated by malignancy. The most commonly encountered is lymphoma, but gastrointestinal carcinomas, usually gastric, also occur. In a series of 205 patients with a variety of primary immunodeficiency diseases, there were three patients with carcinoma of the colon (Spector et al. 1978). Secondary immunodeficiency, usually iatrogenic, is much more common. Among 182 patients who had developed malignancy while receiving immunosuppressive therapy after organ transplantation, there were three who had colorectal cancer (Penn 1974).

Diverticular Disease and Ischaemic Colitis

There is no known association between chronic diverticular disease, or ischaemic colitis, and carcinoma. This is of interest because diverticula in other organs are recognized to be associated with a high incidence of carcinoma in the vicinity, for example in the pharynx, oesophagus, and bladder.

Management Policy for High-Risk Groups of Patients

Although, as indicated above, several chronic inflammatory and immunological diseases of the intestines are associated with carcinoma of the colon, only in ulcerative colitis is there a substantial number of otherwise healthy patients at risk of developing colorectal cancer. Any patient with colitis more extensive than the rectosigmoid should have regular examination of the colon by a double-contrast barium enema or colonoscopy with multiple biopsies, at regular intervals from 10 years after the onset of colitis. If severe epithelial dysplasia is found in colonoscopic biopsies, consideration should be given to prophylactic colectomy. When this is done, some patients will be found already to have developed unrecognized tumours, which may be multiple. When the tumour marker carcinoembryonic antigen (CEA) was identified, it was hoped that serial measurements of this material in serum might be used to screen patients and thus identify early malignancies. Serial studies of CEA have been found to be useless for prediction of the development of malignancy in patients with colitis (Loewenstein and Zamcheck 1978).

In the ulcerative, stricturing diseases such as Crohn's disease, irradiation colitis, and perhaps also chronic infectious diseases, the majority of symptomatic patients will have been treated by resection of the diseased bowel and thus the risk of development of malignancy is substantially reduced. Those patients who have had strictures treated by bypass surgery rather than resection should be carefully observed. Fortunately, improvements in surgical techniques with pre-operative dietary preparation now allow radical surgery to be performed more safely. It is unlikely that many new patients will be added to those at risk with bypassed diseased bowel.

With regard to the possible risk of colorectal cancer in immunodeficiency disease and in coeliac disease, the case must at present be considered 'not proven'. There appears to be no indication for intervention to seek colorectal cancer in these patients.

It is important to emphasize that when considered in the context of colorectal cancer in general, those patients in whom malignancy has developed in a diseased bowel are very much in the minority. For example, in the Gastro-Intestinal Unit at the Western General Hospital, Edinburgh, around 1,000–1,200 new outpatients with gastrointestinal disease are seen annually, and some 25 patients per year are treated for rectal or colonic cancer. It is the policy of the unit to perform a long-term follow-up in patients with malabsorption, ulcerative colitis, and Crohn's disease, but despite this only four patients with carcinoma complicating ulcerative colitis have been seen in the last 6 years. In the same period we have had one patient with coeliac disease and rectal carcinoma (but the coeliac disease was diagnosed by the physician who saw her because of rectal bleeding). Two patients with abdominal tuberculosis and colonic cancer have been mentioned above, and no patient with colonic carcinoma associated with Crohn's disease, immunodeficiency disease, or radiation colitis has been seen.

Immunological Reactions and Colonic Inflammation in Experimental Animals

Despite the considerable research currently being undertaken on carcinogenesis and colon cancers, investigations of the role of the immune system in the pathogenesis of malignancy in the colon has received little attention. For example, in an excellent review on experimental colon cancer (Lamont and O'Gorman 1978), discussion of immunological aspects is confined to reports of work on the host immune responses to tumour-associated antigens. There is now a wealth of information on the nature of the gut-associated lymphoid tissues, and increasing evidence that the gut mucosal T cells play a key role in normal and diseased intestinal mucosal functions. Careful studies of the effects of immunologically mediated damage on the gut, briefly discussed below, have shown that local immune reactions will alter mucosal permeability to macromolecules, and will also influence epithelial cell kinetics by stimulation of crypt mitosis. Thus local antigen-antibody and antigen-lymphocyte interaction deserve further investigation as factors which may potentiate carcinogenesis, although they are unlikely to initiate malignant transformation.

Mucosal T Cells and the Gut-Associated Lymphoid Tissues

There are many T lymphocytes in the organized gut-associated lymphoid tissues such as Peyer's patches and mesenteric lymph nodes, and many T cells are also scattered within the mucosae of the gastrointestinal tract. Mucosal lymphocytes are mainly medium-sized. They are found within the epithelium (intra-epithelial [IE] lymphocytes) and in the lamina propria of the gut (LP lymphocytes). Although the small intestinal mucosa has been most extensively studied, similar IE and LP lymphocytes are present in smaller numbers in gastric and colonic mucosae. Properties of small-bowel IE lymphocytes have been recently reviewed (Ferguson 1977).

Studies in several species, including man, have shown that there are a number of subsets, or subclasses, of T lymphocytes. By the use of various surface markers and tests of function, two principal subsets, *T helper* and *T suppressor,* have been defined. The *T helper* cells secrete lymphokines and are responsible for interaction with B lymphocytes prior to B lymphocyte antibody secretion. The *T suppressor* cells perform various suppressor functions in relation to other T cells, B cells, and macrophages, and are the effector cytotoxic cells for cell-mediated immunity. Studies in the mouse (G. Grand, personal communication) and in man (Selby et al. 1981) have shown that the majority of IE T cells in the small bowel are of the suppressor/cytotoxic phenotype. It is likely that many of the LP lymphocytes are of the *T helper* subclass although antisera to identify this group of cells are more difficult to work with.

We have proposed (Mowat and Ferguson 1981) that this segregation of T cells within the intestinal mucosa has important functional effects. Lamina propria lymphocytes will secrete lymphokines after interaction with antigen (see below), whereas the function of IE lymphocytes will be to suppress immune reactions within the 30 μm deep monolayer of the intestinal mucosal epithelium. It is also possible that the cytotoxic functions of IE lymphocytes confer resistance to malignant disease of the epithelium.

Table 2. Animal models of colonic mucosal hypersensitivity reactions

Type of hypersensitivity	Experimental system	Results	Reference
Reaginic	Man: passive anaphylaxis	Transient oedema mucus secretion	Ferguson 1975
Immune complex	Rabbit: immune complexes I–V local rectal inflammation induced with formalin enema	Acute colitis (polymorph infiltrate epithelium abnormal)	Hodgson et al. 1978
	Rabbit: immune complexes I–V and formalin enema animals previously immunised with with enterobacterial antigen	Acute and chronic colitis (crypt abscesses, bifid glands)	Mee et al. 1979
T cell-mediated	Mice: rejection of heterotransplanted colonic allografts	Lymphocyte infiltrate, epithelium abnormal increased crypt mitotis	Holden and Ferguson 1976, 1979
	Rabbit: skin sensitised to DNCB; challenge by intrarectal DNCB	Ulcers, crypt abscesses (later developed CMI to rabbit colon extracts)	Rabin and Rogers 1978

Effects of Local Immune Reactions on Intestinal Mucosa

Hypersensitivity, antibody-mediated or cell-mediated, is defined as the state of the previously immunized person or animal in which tissue damage results from the immune reaction to a further dose of antigen. Thus there are two stages in any immune-mediated intestinal inflammatory state, induction of immunity involving either antibodies or lymphocytes, and subsequent tissue damage on re-exposure to antigen. The substances concerned may be micro-organisms, parasites, dietary antigens, or autoantigens, or may be unknown (as in the idiopathic chronic inflammatory bowel diseases). It is important to emphasize that although the hypersensitivity reaction may be triggered by specific immunological interaction, effects on the tissue are mediated by various non-specific effector mechanisms. These include the soluble factors produced by lymphocytes, activated polymorphonuclear leukocytes or macrophages, and various direct membrane effects between immune cells and antigen. In addition, specific immune reactions affect several non-immunological intestinal components such as blood flow, motility, mucous secretion, and cell proliferation kinetics of the epithelium.

Many animal experiments have been performed, in which various types of immunological reaction have been used to study the intestinal mucosa, and most work has been concerned with the small intestine (Ferguson and Mowat 1980). The limited work on hypersensitivity reactions in the colon (summarized in Table 2) show similar features.

Reaginic Hypersensitivity

Reaginic hypersensitivity involving IgE antibodies and mast cells rarely results in histopathological change in the mucosa, but leads to a considerable increase in mucosal permeability to macromolecules in both directions between the lumen and the lamina propria. For example, Bloch et al. (1979) showed a greatly increased uptake of immunoreactive bovine serum albumin (a marker protein) from the gut lumen into venous blood when rats were subjected to mild systemic anaphylaxis. Theoretically, reaginic hypersensitivity could increase mucosal permeability to carcinogens of a wide range of molecular size.

Immune Complex Hypersensitivity

The most interesting work in this respect is that of Hodgson's group (Hodgson et al. 1978; Mee et al. 1979), who used the Auer technique to produce immune complex-mediated damage in rabbit colon. Immune complexes, formed in antigen excess, were given intravenously to the rabbits and the complexes were induced to localize in the rectum by mild trauma (produced by rectal instillation of dilute formalin). Both acute and chronic colitis were achieved, and although no formal studies of epithelial cell proliferation were performed, abnormally short and bifid glands were present months after the immune complex damage (Mee et al. 1979).

T Cell-Mediated Immune Reactions

In the rabbit, skin sensitization with a contact sensitizing agent DNCB and intrarectal DNCB challenge were used to produce ulceration, crypt abscesses, and a chronic proctitis (Rabin and Rogers 1978). In our own work we have used mice, and have studied the effects of T cell-mediated immune reactions on the histopathology and epithelial cell kinetics of the small and large bowel. From our work in the small bowel we have proposed that the secretion of lymphokines by activated T cells is the likely mechanism for T cell-mediated intestinal damage with crypt hyperplasia, villous atrophy, and lymphocyte infiltrate (Ferguson and MacDonald 1977). Parallel experiments on the colon, in an experimental model in which fetal colon is transplanted heterotopically into syngenic and allogenic hosts, has shown that the cell-mediated immune reaction of allograft rejection produces a substantial increase in crypt mitotic activity in colonic mucosa prior to destruction of the allografts (Holden and Ferguson 1976, 1979).

Many factors other than cellular immune reactions will influence colonic epithelial cell proliferation, and these include the amount of fibre in the diet, local hormones, nutritional status, and exposure to carcinogens. Clearly there is considerable scope for research on the facilitation of carcinogenesis by mucosal inflammatory reactions, by combining conventional experimental schedules on colon carcinogenesis with induction of mucosal cell-mediated immunity, e.g., by graft-versus-host disease.

Acknowledgments. We are grateful to Dr. W. Sircus and Mr. A. N. Smith for permission to publish details of a patient in their care.

References

Black WC, Ackerman LV (1965) Carcinoma of the large intestine as a late complication of pelvic radiotherapy. Clin Radiol 16: 278–281

Bloch KJ, Bloch DB, Stearns M, Walker WA (1979) Intestinal uptake of macromolecules. VI. Uptake of protein antigen in vivo in normal rats and in rats injected with *Nippostrongylus brasiliensis* or subjected to mild systemic anaphylaxis. Gastroenterology 77: 1039–1044

Bonnevie O, Binder V, Anthonisen P, Riis P (1974) The prognosis of ulcerative colitis. Scand J Gastroenterol 9: 81–91

Butt JH, Lennard-Jones JE, Ritchie JK (1980) A practical approach to the risk of cancer in inflammatory bowel disease. Med Clin North Am 64: 1203–1220

Castro EB, Rosen PP, Quan SHQ (1973) Carcinoma of large intestine in patients irradiated for carcinoma of cervix and uterus. Cancer 31: 45–52

Darke SG, Parks AG, Grogono JL, Pollock DJ (1973) Adenocarcinoma and Crohn's disease. Br J Surg 60: 169–175

de Dombal FT, Waits JMcK, Watkinson G, Goligher JC (1966) Local complications of ulcerative colitis: Structure, pseudopolyposis and carcinoma of colon and rectum. Br Med J 1: 1442–1447

Devroede GJ, Taylor WF, Sauer WG, Jackman RJ, Gunnar BS (1971) Cancer risk and life expectancy of children with ulcerative colitis. N Engl J Med 285: 17–21

Diamond MP, Yardley JH, Bayless TM, Roberts J (1978) Colon carcinoma and severe epithelial dysplasia in patients with ulcerative colitis. (Abstract) Gastroenterology 74: 1120

Dobbins WO (1977) Current status of the precancer lesion in ulcerative colitis. Gastroenterology 73: 1431–1433

Evans DJ, Pollock DJ (1972) In-situ and invasive carcinoma of the colon in patients with ulcerative colitis. Gut 13: 566–570
Ferguson A (1975) Allergy in the gastro-intestinal tract. (Leading article) Lancet 2: 1021–1023
Ferguson A (1977) Intraepithelial lymphocytes of the small intestine. Gut 18: 921–937
Ferguson A, MacDonald TT (1977) Effects of local delayed hypersensitivity on the small intestine. In: Ciba Foundation Symposium no. 46. Elsevier/North-Holland, Amsterdam, pp 305–327
Ferguson A, Mowat AMcI (1980) Immunological mechanisms in the small intestine. In: Wright R (ed) Recent advances in gastrointestinal pathology. Saunders, Eastbourne, pp 93–103
Gilat T, Zemishlany Z, Ribak J, Benaroya Y, Lilos P (1974) Ulcerative colitis in the Jewish population of Tel Aviv. Yafo II. The rarity of malignant degeneration. Gastroenterology 67: 933–938
Greenstein AJ, Sachar DB, Pucillo A, Kreel I, Geller S, Janowitz HD, Aufses A (1978) Cancer in Crohn's disease after diversionary surgery. Am J Surg 135: 86–90
Greenstein AJ, Sachar DB, Smith H, Pucillo A, Papatestas AE, Kreel I, Geller SA, Janowitz HD, Aufses AH (1979) Cancer in universal and left-sided ulcerative colitis: Factors determining risk. Gastroenterology 77: 290–294
Gyde SN, Prior P, Macartney JC, Thompson H, Waterhouse JAH, Allan RN (1980) Malignancy in Crohn's disease. Gut 21: 1024–1029
Harris OD, Cooke WT, Thompson H, Waterhouse JAH (1967) Malignancy in adult coeliac disease and idiopathic steatorrhoea. Am J Med 42: 899–912
Hodgson HJF, Potter BJ, Skinner J, Jewell DP (1978) Immune complex mediated colitis in rabbits. An experimental model. Gut 19: 225–232
Holden RJ, Ferguson A (1976) Histopathology of a cell mediated immune reaction in mouse colon – allograft rejection. Gut 17: 661–670
Holden RJ, Ferguson A (1979) Effects of age, antigen deprivation and allograft rejection on epithelial cell kinetics in mouse colon. Gut 20: 234–239
Holmes GKT, Stokes PL, Sorahan TM, Prior P, Waterhouse JAH, Cooke WT (1976) Coeliac disease, gluten-free diet and malignancy. Gut 17: 612–619
Kewenter J, Ahlman H, Hulten L (1978) Cancer risk in extensive ulcerative colitis. Ann Surg 188: 824–828
Lamont JT, O'Gorman TA (1978) Experimental colon cancer. Gastroenterology 75: 1157–1169
Lennard-Jones JE, Morson BC, Ritchie JK, Shove DC, Williams CB (1977) Cancer in colitis: Assessment of the individual risk by clinical and histological criteria. Gastroenterology 73: 1280–1289
Lightdale CJ, Sternberg SS, Posner G, Sherlock P (1975) Carcinoma complicating Crohn's disease. Am J Med 59: 262–268
Loewenstein MS, Zamcheck N (1978) Carcinoembryonic antigen (CEA) levels in benign gastrointesinal disease states. Cancer 42: 1412–1418
Mee AS, McLaughlin JE, Hodgson HJF, Jewell DP (1979) Chronic immune colitis in rabbits. Gut 20: 1–5
Ming-Chai C, Jen-Chun H, P'ei-Yu C, Ch'i-Yuan C, P'eng-Fei T, Shen-Hsing C, Fu-P'an W, Ts'u-Ling C, Shun-Chuan C (1965) Pathogenesis of carcinoma of the colon and rectum in *Schistosomiasis japonica*. Chin Med J 84: 513–525
Morson BC, Pang SC (1967) Rectal biopsy as an aid to cancer control in ulcerative colitis. Gut 8: 423–434
Mowat AMcI, Ferguson A (1981) Induction and expression of mucosal cell-mediated immunity. In: Bourne FJ (ed) Current topics in veterinary medicine and animal science. Martinus Nijhoff, London
Nedbal J, Maratka Z (1968) Ulcerative proctocolitis in Czechoslovakia. Am J Proctol 19: 106–114

Penn I (1974) Occurrence of cancer in immune deficiencies. Cancer 34: 858–866
Rabin BS, Rogers SJ (1978) A cell-mediated immune model of inflammatory bowel disease in the rabbit. Gastroenterology 75: 29–33
Renton P, Blackshaw AJ (1976) Colonic lymphoma complicating ulcerative colitis. Br J Surg 63: 542–545
Riddell RH, Morson BC (1979) Value of sigmoidoscopy and biopsy in the detection of carcinoma and premalignant change in ulcerative colitis. Gut 20: 575–580
Selby WS, Janossy G, Jewell DP (1981) Immunohistological characterisation of intra-epithelial lymphocytes of the human gastrointestinal tract. Gut 22: 169–176
Slaney G (1971) Results of treatment of carcinoma of the colon and rectum. In: Irvine WT (ed) Modern trends in surgery, vol 3. Butterworths, London, pp 69–89
Spector DB, Good RA, Kersey JH (1978) Immunodeficiency diseases and malignancy. In: Lipkin M, Good RA (eds) Gastrointestinal tract cancer. Plenum Press, New York London, pp 51–70
Weedon DD, Shorter RG, Ilstrup DM, Huizenga KA, Taylor WF (1973) Crohn's disease and cancer. N Engl J Med 289: 1099–1103
Yardley JH, Keren DF (1974) 'Precancer' lesions in ulcerative colitis. A retrospective study of rectal biopsy and colectomy specimens. Cancer 34: 835–844

Genetic Factors

H. J. R. Bussey

Department of Pathology, St. Mark's Hospital, London EC1V 2PS, United Kingdom

The large intestine is one of the major sites for malignant disease in man, being in this respect second only to the lungs. About 16,500 persons die annually from colorectal cancer in England and Wales, and the tendency is for this figure to rise slowly. Considerable research has been directed at the problem of reducing thc incidence of the disease and one of the main targets investigated has been the possibility that differences in environmental factors, such as diet and social habits, may be related to the variable incidence of colorectal cancer in different regions of the world. Any attempt to explain the aetiology of colorectal cancer cannot ignore what histopathological studies have revealed about the close relationship between intestinal adenomas and cancers. Moreover, such an attempt must also take into consideration the facts revealed by studies of the rare and interesting condition known as 'familial polyposis coli'. Not only is it the outstanding example of the adenoma-carcinoma sequence, but it also introduces an irrefutable genetic factor into the problem.

Familial Polyposis Coli

There is no evidence that colorectal cancer is inherited but there is evidence that some precancerous conditions have a genetic origin. The most notable example is familial polyposis coli (Bussey 1975). This is a condition affecting the gastrointestinal tract, but mainly the large intestine, and has three main features:
1) The presence of numerous adenomatous polyps,
2) a high incidence of associated colorectal cancer,
3) a genetic origin.

The adenomas seldom number less than 500 and may sometimes exceed 5,000, when the mucosa is so covered with the tumours that it is difficult to see normal mucosa between them. The average number in colectomy specimens resected for polyposis is about 1,000 and the tumours are generally fairly evenly distributed around the colorectum. In the early stages of the disease, the lesions are flat mucosal nodules measuring up to 5 mm in diameter which do not give rise to any symptoms. In the majority of cases the polyps will have begun to appear in the large intestine by the age of 20 years, but on average it will be another 10 years before symptoms appear. These begin with gradually increasing bowel movements, mucous discharge, and occasional episodes of bleeding from the rectum. By this time many of the polyps will exceed 1 cm in diameter and will have developed long stalks (Fig. 1). It is usual for the larger polyps to be found in the descending and sigmoid segments of the colon and in the rectum.

Recent Results in Cancer Research, Vol. 83

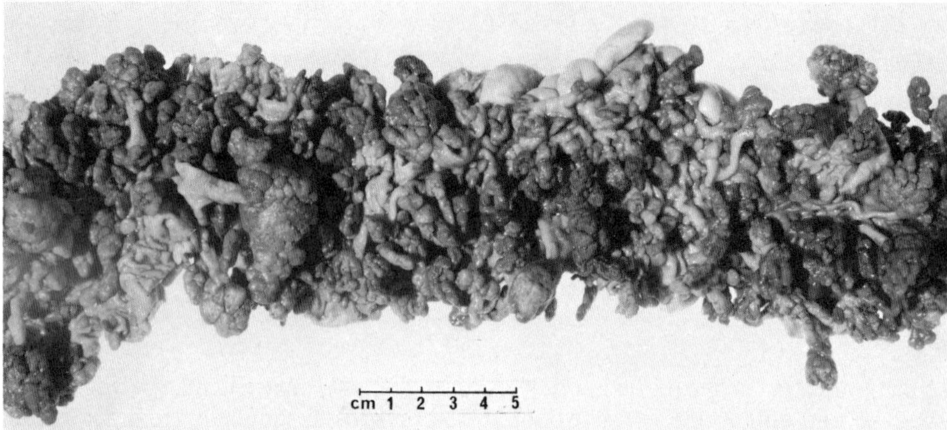

Fig. 1. Portion of colectomy specimen showing numerous large pedunculated adenomas

The insidious onset of the symptoms is often ignored until persistent severe bloody diarrhoea forces the patient to seek advice and the diagnois is made.

It is at this point that the second characteristic of polyposis coli is usually encountered. No less than two-thirds of the patients presenting with symptoms are found on investigation already to have cancer of the colon or rectum. The only effective treatment for polyposis is surgery, either by removal of the whole large intestine, necessitating an ileostomy, or by resection of the colon only, continuity of the bowel being restored by ileorectal anastomosis. The rectal adenomas are destroyed by diathermy treatment, but regular surveillance of the rectum at about 6-monthly intervals is necessary to deal with any new adenomas which may develop. These operations were not available before World War II, and until about 1950 patients with polyposis were not generally operated upon until cancer supervened. The records of the St Mark's Hospital Polyposis Register in the pre-colectomy period indicate that about 90% of the polyposis patients eventually developed colorectal cancer at an average age of just over 40 years, which is about 30 years younger than that for the general population. There was no guarantee that the remainder would have escaped the same fate had they lived longer. The probability, therefore, of an untreated patient not developing intestinal malignancy is very slight.

The third feature of polyposis is found when the family history is investigated. Cripps (1882) recorded polyposis in two patients who were brother and sister, and this is accepted as the first report of its familial occurrence. Since then, numerous families have been studied (the St Mark's Hospital Polyposis Register currently contains 265 families) and it has been established beyond doubt that polyposis coli is a genetic disorder inherited as an autosomal dominant characteristic (Fig. 2). With each new patient found to have the condition, it is important to construct a family pedigree unless this is already known. Since every child of a polyposis patient has a 50-50 chance of inheriting polyposis, a list can be compiled of all family members at risk, who should be alerted and advised to seek examination. Children are checked by sigmoidoscopic examination performed first around the age of 14 years and repeated, if negative, at intervals of 1–2 years. This policy has resulted in a reduction in the incidence of associated colorectal cancer from 66% in the patients presenting with symptoms to

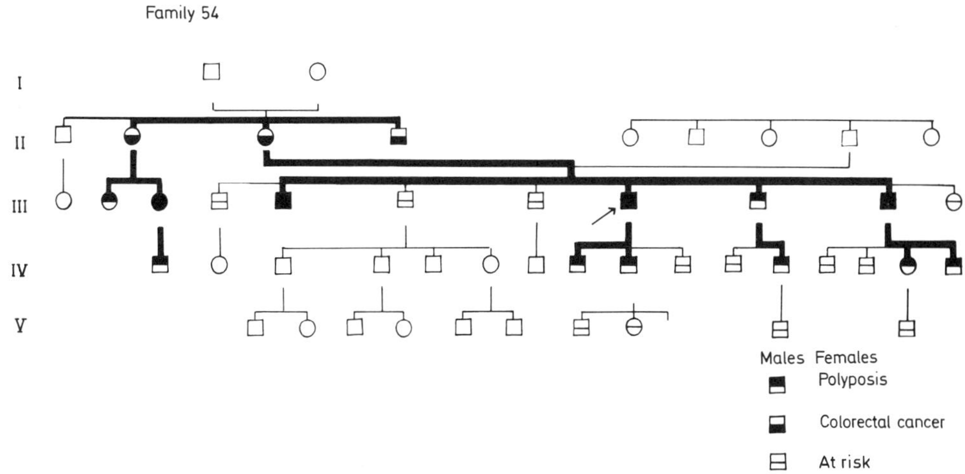

Fig. 2. Pedigree of typical polyposis family. The pattern of inheritance is traced by the *thick line*. Only affected members can pass on the condition, which is inherited by approximately one-half of their children

about 5% in those called up for examination because they were known to be at risk.

Familial Polyposis as a Working Model

Polyposis coli has received little attention from workers concerned with the problem of colorectal cancer, and it is generally regarded as a freak condition–interesting, but with little to offer that is helpful towards a solution. It is true that the contribution that polyposis makes to the sum total of colorectal cancer in the community is trivial (perhaps only 100 cases annually out of nearly 17,000) but the condition itself is really a microcosm in which the main constituents of the problem can be studied. The multiplicity of adenomas and a high incidence of associated cancer afford opportunities of following the development of adenomas from the earliest stages through to malignant degeneration such as are not easily available elsewhere. The fact that a genetic factor is involved is something that must be taken into account in any explanation of the aetiology of colorectal cancer. That the condition is inherited also ensures that a pool of individuals is available for the investigation of factors that might affect polyposis, the results of which, if advantageous, might well be applied with equal success to the much larger problem of colorectal cancer in the general population.

Polyposis coli is thus a useful experimental model providing considerable support for the adenoma-carcinoma sequence, which is discussed later. There is, for instance, the direct evidence of cancer developing in adenomatous polyps, the incidence of which in polyposis cases is about one-third of all cancers (Bussey 1975). Again, polyposis is not only the condition with the highest incidence of associated malignancy, but also one in which multiple colorectal cancers are most frequent, being found in about one-half of the cases.

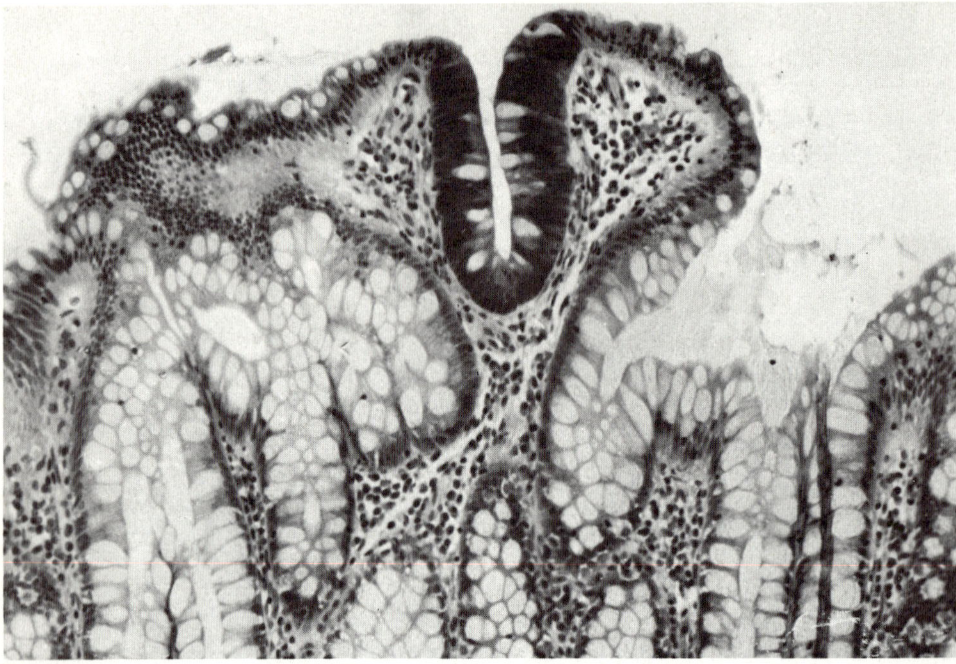

Fig. 3. A small area of epithelial dysplasia within a single tubule of the colonic mucosa. The increased density of the epithelial cells, nuclear hyperchromatism, and loss of mucin production indicate an early stage in the formation of an adenoma. × 180

The possibility of studying the histopathological evolution of intestinal adenomas has been mentioned. It does not require many colectomy specimens removed for polyposis to observe the sequence of stages from the single tubule lined with dysplastic epithelium (Fig. 3) to the mature adenoma (Bussey 1979).

Another aspect of polyposis, which it is suggested may be of fundamental importance to the whole problem of colorectal cancer, is that of inheritance. Polyposis raises questions as to what exactly is inherited – cancer, adenomas or just a 'proneness' to produce adenomas – how far other factors, genetic or environmental, are involved at different stages, and to what extent these factors apply to the adenomas of non-polyposis patients. To find answers to these questions it is necessary to look in more detail at the nature of adenomas and cancers of the large intestine and the relationship between them.

Histopathology of Intestinal Adenomas and Carcinomas

Adenomas of the colorectum are derived from the mucus-secreting epithelium lining the large intestine. They consist of masses of epithelium showing abnormal growth patterns to which histopathologists apply the term 'dysplasia'. The dysplasia may be subdivided at histological level into mild, moderate, or severe as the growth pattern increasingly differs from that of the normal epithelium (Muto et al. 1975) (Figs. 4–6). Adenomas may also be subdivided into tubular and villous types. These are not strictly

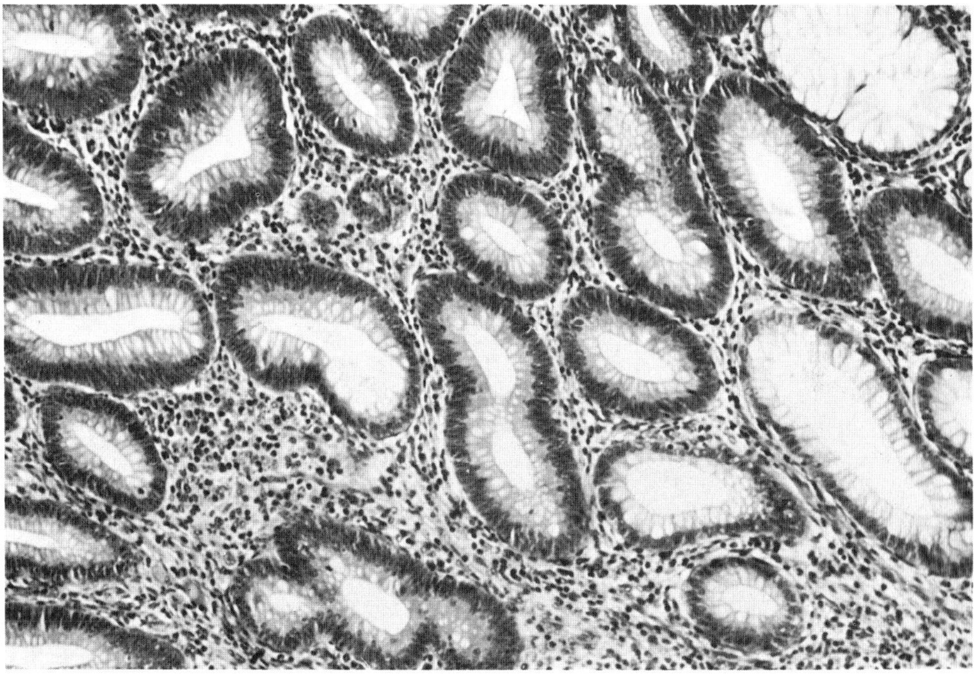

Fig. 4. Mild epithelial dysplasia. Compared with the normal tubules on the *right,* the more closely packed cells are beginning to show stratification but the size and arrangement of glands are little altered. × 150

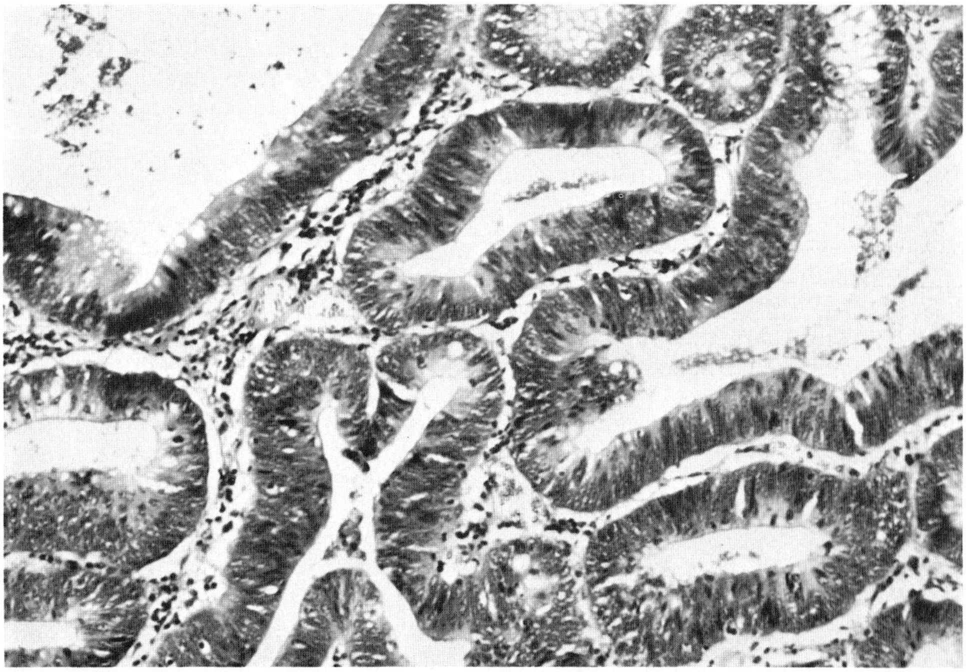

Fig. 5. Moderate epithelial dysplasia. The tubules are distorted and tortuous and the lining cells more stratified but retaining polarity in most regions. × 150

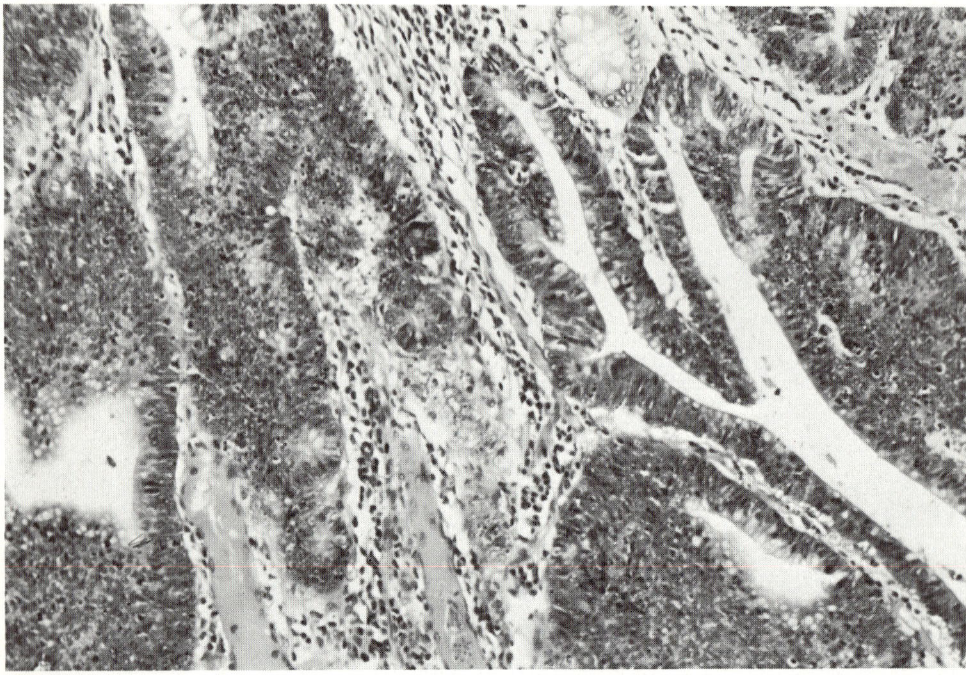

Fig. 6. Severe epithelial dysplasia. Further loss of glandular pattern with increased disorientation of the epithelial cells with back-to-back arrangement and intraglandular bridging of the tubules. Almost complete absence of mucin. × 150

different entities, but rather opposite ends of a spectrum connected by the intermediate tubulovillous adenoma. The microscopical appearances of the two types are reflected in their morphology. The tubular adenoma (or adenomatous polyp) is usually a pedunculated nodular tumour and the villous adenoma is a sessile broad-based shaggy growth (Morson and Dawson 1979).

When cancer of the large intestine is discussed it is the malignant tumour of the adenocarcinomatous type which is usually considered. Adenocarcinomas account for about 99% of the total malignant tumours of the colorectum, the other 1% being composed mainly of leiomyosarcomas and lymphomas. The adenocarcinomas, like the adenomas, are derived from the intestinal mucus-secreting epithelium. They show varying degrees of dysplasia and have a further characteristic of abnormal growth, namely invasion of the adjacent normal tissues. The common factor of disorderly growth, though perhaps in different degrees, has been one reason for suspecting a close relationship between adenomas and carcinomas. This relationship has been investigated in detail in recent years (Enterline et al. 1962; Morson 1974; Muto et al. 1975) and because of its importance in the aetiology of colorectal cancer has come to be called the 'adenoma-carcinoma sequence'.

The Adenoma-Carcinoma Sequence

The most direct evidence that adenomas play a part in the genesis of colorectal cancer is the actual observation of cancer developing within an adenomatous tumour. That

this is not an uncommon occurrence is indicated in a report by Muto et al. (1975) that of 1961 intestinal cancers investigated, 278 (14.2%) revealed evidence of residual adenoma at the periphery of the carcinoma. Morson (1974) studied a different series of 2,305 colorectal cancers, in which the corresponding figure for contiguous benign tumour was 10.7%. The cases were divided into three subgroups in which the invasion of the cancer (1) was limited to the submucosa; (2) extended into the muscle coat but not beyond; and (3) extended through the bowel wall into the surrounding tissues. The incidence of contiguous adenoma in the three groups was found to be 56.6%, 18.3%, and 7.6%, respectively. The inference is that as the cancer expands, the original adenoma in which the malignancy developed is progressively destroyed. This view is supported by other evidence. Approximately 4% of patients with colorectal cancer have multiple synchronous intestinal cancers. In these tumours the proportion found to show evidence of origin in an adenoma was 27.0%, or double that observed among cancers occurring singly (Heald and Bussey 1975). The difference is greater still among polyposis patients with associated colorectal cancer. About half these patients have multiple synchronous cancers, and among these the incidence of contiguous adenoma is 36%. When multiple cancers are present they are usually at different stages of advancement. The symptoms due to the more advanced tumours result in discovery of the less advanced cancers at a stage when the initiating adenoma is less eroded.
Further evidence for the adenoma-carcinoma sequence is provided by studying the incidence of associated colorectal cancer in patients with differing numbers of adenomas. In the series of patients investigated by Muto et al. (1975) there were 1,582 with adenomas, 439 of whom (27.7%) had associated colorectal cancer. A break-down of the series into groups with varying numbers of adenomas showed that there was a direct relationship between the number of adenomas and the incidence of associated malignancy (Table 1). It has already been mentioned that familial polyposis coli is the condition in which the greatest number of adenomas occurs and which also has the highest incidence of colorectal cancer.
It is obvious that the relationship between adenomas and cancers is one of considerable importance. In fact, as the evidence accumulates, it is difficult to avoid the conclusion that most, perhaps even all, cancers of the colon and rectum originate in pre-existing adenomas. The converse, however, is not true. There is no evidence that, given time, all adenomas become cancerous, though it may be that the potential is inherent in all of them. The subsequent development of malignancy is almost certainly dependent on other factors of an environmental nature.

Adenomas and Carcinomas in Polyposis and Non-Polyposis Patients

Evidence has been produced for the validity of the adenoma-carcinoma sequence and for the essential role played by adenomas in the aetiology of colorectal cancer. It is important to decide what differences, if any, exist between the adenomas of polyposis coli and those occurring in the non-polyposis patient. One obvious difference is that of number. It has been stated that in polyposis the average number of adenomas is about 1,000, the range being generally between 400 and 4,000, although occasionally counts down to 150 and up to 5,000 have been recorded. In non-polyposis patients there are usually fewer than 20 adenomas, though in rare instances up to 80 or so may be present. The figure of 100 adenomas is a practical one to use as a division between the two groups of patients.

Table 1. Relationship of number of adenomas and incidence of associated carcinoma

Number of adenomas	1	2	3	4	5	6 or more	Polyposis (1,000)
Number of patients	1,199	249	66	40	12	16	–
Number with cancer	263	106	30	20	9	11	–
Percentage with cancer	21.9	42.6	45.5	50.0	75.0	68.8	(90 +)

The early stages in the development of adenomas in polyposis are the presence of single tubules lined with dysplastic epithelium and of micro-adenomas composed of small groups of such tubules (Bussey 1979). Similar changes have been observed in small numbers in a series of specimens from non-polyposis cancer cases (Oohara et al. 1979). It appears that the developmental process is similar for all adenomas. The scarcity of foci of dysplasia from which adenomas can result is the only reason why the process is infrequently seen in non-polyposis patients.

The various histopathological types of adenomas (tubular, villous, and tubulovillous) are found in both groups, and in approximately similar proportions. Gibbs (1967) found the incidence and density of argentaffin and Paneth cells to be the same in tubular and villous adenomas from both polyposis and non-polyposis patients.

Finally, a comparison of the carcinomas associated with polyposis and those occurring in the general population shows few differences. The proportions of Dukes' stages and of the different histological grades of malignancy, the site distribution in the large intestine, and the 5-year survival rates are substantially the same. An increase in the proportion of cancers in polyposis with contiguous adenoma has already been explained as the result of an increase in the number of polyposis patients with multiple synchronous colorectal cancers. The average age at diagnosis of intestinal cancer in polyposis patients is about 40 years, which is some 25 years younger than in the general population. This is obviously connected with the correspondingly earlier appearance of the adenomas, although the factors controlling this are not known. To sum up the evidence so far, it is probable that there is no significant difference between adenomas and carcinomas in polyposis and non-polyposis patients other than that of number. However, one other factor, that of possible inheritance, remains to be investigated.

At this stage, the following points can be listed:

1) Intestinal adenomas occur in both polyposis and non-polyposis patients, although in much larger numbers in the former group;
2) No difference has been detected between the histological and clinical characteristics of the adenomas occurring in the two groups;
3) In both polyposis and non-polyposis patients, adenomas are the main and possibly the only precursor of intestinal malignancy. The resulting cancers show similar characteristics;
4) In polyposis coli the adenomas result from genetic mutation.

The question which naturally arises is whether, in view of all the other similarities in the adenomas in the two groups, it is not possible that the adenomas in non-polyposis patients may also have a genetic origin.

Are All Adenomas Genetic in Origin?

This possibility was first suggested by Woolf et al. (1955). They had investigated a family with a high incidence of intestinal cancer and also found polyps, in small numbers, in a large proportion of family members. It was thought that the increase in colorectal cancer might be due to inheritance of the polyps. No conclusion was reached as to the mechanism of the inheritance, and it is unfortunate that the pathology does not identify the polyps as adenomas but only as being 'simple' or 'hyperplastic' in nature.

Veale (1965) came to the conclusion that all intestinal adenomas were genetic in origin and that those occurring in non-polyposis patients were a Mendelian recessive characteristic. He had analysed data from the St Mark's Hospital Polyposis Register and from a large polyposis family investigated in New Zealand. Certain anomalies suggested that the material was made up from two components, one being perhaps due to the polyposis gene being modified by another mutated gene. Veale postulated that the normal wild gene (+) at a certain position in a chromosome could undergo two types of mutation. The first mutation (P) would result in the inheritance of familial polyposis coli. The second mutation (p) would also give rise to adenomas, but would differ from P in that the adenomas would be few in number and the inheritance would be of a Mendelian recessive nature. If this hypothesis is correct, the possible genotypes for polyposis would be P+ and Pp. Polyposis would result in either case because of the presence of P, but when this was associated with p Veale thought there might be an earlier and more severe onset of the condition. It is certainly easy to find examples that clinically differ sufficiently to support this idea, but this does not rule out other possible explanations, such as environmental factors. The concept of a gene mutation of the p type, producing few adenomas as a recessive characteristic, proved worthy of investigation. Here the three possible genotypes would be:

1) ++ Individuals with this genotype would be homozygous for the normal or wild gene and would not develop adenomas;
2) p+ Heterozygous individuals, who almost certainly would not be adenoma-prone;
3) pp Patients with this genotype would be capable of producing adenomas. Investigations indicate that in general the number of adenomas is likely to be less than 10, and only rarely more than 50.

At the time that Veale suggested this hypothesis there was little supportative evidence. There were a few reports of families with unusually large numbers of members with colorectal cancer, but apart from the report published by Woolf et al. (1955), there were few references to the presence of polyps. At present, with the adenoma-carcinoma sequence in mind, it is the adenoma which should be the prior objective of any investigation of genetic factors in colorectal cancer. It has to be admitted, however, that the study of the familial incidence of adenomas poses considerable difficulties, which will be discussed later. For the moment, the evidence for the existence of what are generally termed colorectal cancer families will be reviewed.

Colorectal Cancer Families

From time to time reports have been published of families in which the incidence of colorectal cancer among family members is sufficiently high to excite comment

(Mathis 1962; Kluge 1964; Lynch and Krush 1967; Dunstone and Knaggs 1972; Lovett 1976a). Systematic investigations of the family histories of patients with colorectal cancer are less frequently reported. An increase over the expected incidence of intestinal cancer was found by Macklin (1960) when she investigated the family histories of 145 patients who had undergone surgery for the condition. No simple pattern of inheritance emerged from the study to account for the increased incidence.

A more detailed study of a large series was carried out by Lovett (1976b). Satisfactory family histories were obtained from a total of 209 patients admitted to St Mark's Hospital with cancer of the colon or rectum. Lovett found that death certificates of first-degree relatives showed an increase in the observed incidence of colorectal cancer, to about three times the expected figure in the case of parents and about five times the expected figure for brothers and sisters. About one-quarter of the index patients had adenomas as well as cancer in the resected specimen and just under one-third of the patients with adenomas had a positive family history. Although Lovett did not state what proportion of the families had multiple members with colorectal cancer, a subsequent review of her material showed that more than a quarter of the index patients had other affected relatives (Table 2).

The variability of the incidence of colorectal cancer in different families and the contradictory views as to whether or not the inheritance is dominant or recessive are difficult to explain. They may be better understood if the results of various

Table 2. Number of family members with colorectal cancer

Number of family members with colorectal cancer	Total cancer cases	Number of families	
Index cases only	1	154	
Index case + 1 relative	2	48	26.3%
Index case + 2 relatives	3	4	
Index case + 3 relatives	4	3	

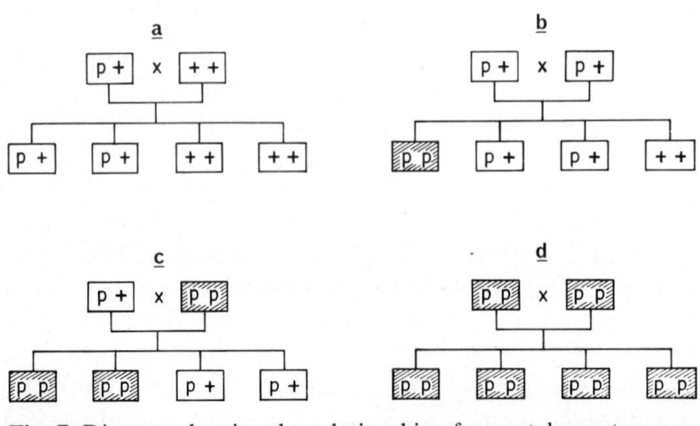

Fig. 7. Diagram showing the relationship of parental genotypes and the incidence of colorectal adenomas in the family

combinations of the genotypes are considered on the assumption that the adenomas are a recessive characteristic. Four possibilities are illustrated in Fig. 7. In the first type (a) no adenoma producers are involved. With two heterozygous parents, as in (b), one-quarter of the children are homozygous and, therefore, adenoma-prone. The third example (c) indicates that half the offspring are adenoma producers, being homozygous, and half will not produce adenomas. Finally, in type (d) all family members are adenoma-prone. In such families, particularly where there are numerous children and conditions are favourable for malignant degeneration within the adenomas, the incidence of colorectal cancer could be high. In fact, its incidence may be so high that it appears to be the result of a dominant inheritance.

It might be thought that matings of the last two types must be exceedingly uncommon, but this depends upon the frequency of the p gene in the general population. This can be estimated from the proportion of adenoma producers in the population, which is not known precisely but for which Veale accepted a figure of about 9%; this gives a frequency for the p gene of around 30%. The proportions of the three genotypes in the community would then be:

++ 49%
p+ 42%
pp 9%.

In other words, half the population have at least one p gene and the changes of unions of the pp × p+ and the pp × pp types are of the order of 1 in 13 and 1 in 125, respectively. Finally, it is possible to make a rough estimate of the chances of adenoma producers developing cancer. Approximately 3% of the population suffer from cancer of the colon or rectum. Since the incidence of adenoma-prone individuals is considered to be about 9%, the likelihood of their developing cancer is presumably 1 in 3. Recent analysis has suggested a slightly lower probability of 1 in 4 becoming malignant, which may reflect either an underestimate of the incidence of adenomas in the population or an overestimate of that of intestinal cancer.

Difficulties in Determining the Inheritance of Adenomas

The greater awareness of familial intestinal cancer has resulted in an increase in the number of examples being brought to notice. Investigation of these families from the genetic aspect and with a view to the possible estimation of the variable risk attached to individual members has revealed difficulties not encountered when dealing with polyposis families. Polyposis coli is now established as an autosomal dominant characteristic. The expected pattern of inheritance is known and it is usually easy to identify the family members at risk. In colorectal cancer families, a genetic factor is a possibility that has yet to acquire the degree of certainty attached to polyposis. If Veale's hypothesis is correct and the factor is of the recessive type, the accumulation of evidence supporting a genetic origin for all adenomas is likely to be a slow and complex process. There are several reasons for making this statement. It is necessary, for instance, to investigate the family history of both parents of any colorectal cancer patient: nor must that of the spouse be omitted if the risk to the children is to be estimated. Thus more history taking is involved than with polyposis families and a less complete picture of the family incidence of pp genotypes is likely to emerge. In the absence of any known marker for this genotype, its presence is only indicated by the presence of adenomas or cancers, and in general it is only the latter which are revealed by the family history. The adenomas may have to be searched for and this is more difficult than in polyposis families, where the members at risk are more clearly defined and the adenomas numerous enough to be diagnosed by sigmoidoscopic examination. With non-polyposis patients, investigation of the whole colon by barium enema or colonoscopic examination is necessary. Both are more time-consuming and expensive than sigmoidoscopy. A negative examination does not necessarily exclude either the P or the pp genotype, as the adenomas may develop subsequently, but this is more likely to occur in the non-polyposis patients. In most patients polyposis will have been diagnosed by the age of 25 years, and few family members under regular surveillance will develop the condition after 40 years of age. On the other hand, intestinal adenomas and cancers are uncommon before the age of 40 years, the majority being diagnosed after the age of 60 years. In fact, colonic examinations might have to be continued to 80 years or more before confirming that the patient is of the pp genotype! There is another complication connected with colorectal cancer families. In the absence of a marker for the p gene, there is no way of identifying the heterozygous individual (p+) or the increased risk he or she might be conveying to certain of their children (see Fig. 7b and c). There is no doubt that the most urgent need in investigation of the problem of the inheritance of colorectal cancer is the need for a reliable marker for the p gene.

Relationship of Genetic and Environmental Factors

The suggestion has been made that genetic factors may initiate all types of adenomas. It must be emphasized that this is not to devalue the role played by environmental factors in the subsequent development of adenomatous tumours. Their importance is supported by the epidemiological information available about the incidence of adenomas and cancers in different geographical areas. Some features of these tumours, such as their number, size and subsite distribution around the colon, may be correlated with the dietary habits and geographic incidence of colorectal cancer. Subsequent analysis may be used to identify the nature of the factors responsible for the adenoma-carcinoma sequence.

Hill et al. (1978) have combined epidemiological and histopathological data with Veale's genetic hypothesis to suggest the minimal requirements for a model to explain the aetiology of the adenoma-carcinoma sequence. Slightly modified later (Hill 1978), this model postulates a genetic factor (pp) which is acted on by three other environmental factors, E1, E2, and C. E1 causes the formation of small adenomas in the adenoma-prone colonic epithelium of the individual who is of pp or P genotype. The second environmental factor, E2, is necessary for the growth of the adenomas, and C is the carcinogen that induces the change to malignancy within the large adenomas. There is evidence that E2 is probably the bacteria metabolite of the bile acids incriminated in the aetiology of large bowel cancer (Hill et al. 1975).

Prevention of Colorectal Cancer

The practical value of models like that suggested by Hill et al. (1978) is that they indicate stages at which the adenoma-carcinoma sequence might be interrupted. While it may be possible in due course to reverse gene mutations, it is more likely that some degree of cancer prevention will be achieved by the identification and avoidance of the environmental factors involved. At present cancer prevention is being practised in polyposis coli patients by interrupting the progress from adenoma to cancer by surgical removal of the adenomas while they are still small. The knowledge that polyposis is a genetic disease enables those at risk to be identified and this is vital in ensuring that the adenomas are treated at the correct time. The incidence of cancer of the large intestine in polyposis patients has been reduced from more than 90% to arround 10%, with the possibility of further improvement. Unfortunately the effect of this on the incidence of intestinal cancer in the general population is negligible. In the United Kingdom there are probably less than 100 persons born each year who will develop polyposis. Against that figure must be set nearly 17,000 cases annually of non-polyposis cancer. If these also result from the inheritance of adenoma-proneness, it might be possible to exercise some degree of cancer prevention in the general population. It would be necessary to adapt the methods already applied to polyposis patients, of investigating the family members at most risk and destroying the adenomas as they appear.

An attempt to follow-up the families of all colorectal patients would be an enormous task. The available radiological and colonoscopical facilities could, however, be concentrated on the individuals at greatest risk. Family histories would be essential for the selection process. Members of families with a high incidence of colorectal cancer would be obvious targets, but among the family members there are variable degrees of risk. For example, if the only genetic information about a patient is that one parent had intestinal cancer, his risk of developing adenomas at some time in his life can be estimated at a minimum figure of about 30%. If, in addition, one sibling is also known to have suffered from bowel cancer the risk rises to 65%, and if both parents were affected the ultimate development of adenomas can be predicted with virtual certainty.

The present policy at St Mark's Hospital is to keep a check on those individuals considered to be at greatest risk because of the family history or knowledge of previous cancer or adenomas, particularly if the latter were numerous or showed severe dysplasia. These patients usually have repeat barium enema or colonoscopic examinations at intervals of about 3–4 years. Any metachronous adenomas detected are usually removed by endoscopic polypectomy. A small number of carcinomas have also been discovered and dealt with. It is still too early to know what effect this policy will have in reducing the incidence of colorectal cancer, but the initial success in the detection and destruction of asymptomatic adenomas is encouraging.

References

Bussey HJR (1975) Familial polyposis coli. Johns Hopkins University Press, Baltimore London

Bussey HJR (1979) Familial polyposis coli. In: Sommers SC, Rosen PP (eds) Pathology annual, part I, 1979. Appleton-Century-Crofts, New York, pp 61–81

Cripps WH (1882) Two cases of disseminated polyps of the rectum. Trans Pathol Soc Lond 33: 165–168

Dunstone GH, Knaggs TWL (1972) Familial cancer of the colon and rectum. J Med Genet 9: 451–456

Enterline HT, Evans GW, Mercado-Lugo R, Miller L, Fitts WT (1962) Malignant potential of adenomas of the colon and rectum. JAMA 179: 322–330

Gibbs NM (1967) Incidence and significance of argentaffin and Paneth cells in some tumours of the large intestine. J Clin Pathol 20: 826–831
Heald RJ, Bussey HJR (1975) Clinical experiences at St Mark's Hospital with multiple synchronous cancers of the colon and rectum. Dis Colon Rectum 18: 6–10
Hill M (1978) Etiology of the adenoma-carcinoma sequence. In: Morson BC (ed) The pathogenesis of colorectal cancer. Saunders, Philadelphia London Toronto, pp 153–162
Hill MJ, Morson BC, Bussey HJR (1978) Aetiology of adenoma-carcinoma sequence in large bowel. Lancet 1: 245–247
Kluge T (1964) Familial cancer of the colon. Acta Chir Scand 127: 392–398
Lovett E (1976a) Familial cancer of the gastrointestinal tract. Br J Surg 63: 19–22
Lovett E (1976b) Family studies in cancer of the colon and rectum. Br J Surg 63: 13–18
Lynch HT, Krush AJ (1967) Heredity and carcinoma of the colon. Am J Med 53: 517–527
Macklin MT (1960) Inheritance of cancer of the stomach and large intestine in man. J Natl Cancer Inst 24: 551–571
Mathis M (1962) Familial carcinoma of the colon. A family tree from the Canton of Argau. Schweiz Med Wochenschr 92: 1673–1678
Morson BC (1974) The polyp-cancer sequence in the large bowel. Proc R Soc Med 67: 451–457
Morson BC, Dawson IMP (1979) Gastrointestinal pathology, 2nd edn. Blackwell Scientific, Oxford London Edinburgh Melbourne, p 615
Muto T, Bussey HJR, Morson BC (1975) The evolution of cancer of the colon and rectum. Cancer 36: 2251–2270
Oohara T, Ogino A, Saji K, Tohma H (1979) Difference of colonic mucosa as backgrounds of single advanced carcinoma, benign diseases and familial polyposis of the colon. Stomach and Intestine 14: 811–818
Veale AMO (1965) Intestinal polyposis. Cambridge University Press, London (Eugenics Laboratory Memoirs series no. 40)
Woolf CM, Richards RC, Gardner EJ (1955) Occasional discrete polyps of the colon and rectum showing an inherited tendency in a kindred. Cancer 8: 403–408

Pathology and Natural History

I. C. Talbot

Department of Pathology, University of Leicester, Leicester, LE2 YLX, United Kingdom

Genesis of Colorectal Cancer

Despite statements to the contrary (Horn 1971), a great deal of evidence has now been amassed which indicates that carcinoma of the large bowel arises from a pre-existing premalignant lesion, either an adenoma (Day and Morson 1978) or the dysplasia of long-standing ulcerative colitis (Riddell et al. 1978). Muto et al. (1975) found histological evidence of origin in a benign tumour in 14.2% of 1961 cases of colorectal cancer. The incidence of residual benign tumour was particularly high (56.6%) in early carcinomas confined to the submucosa, suggesting that as a tumour enlarges and invades deeper into the bowel wall the evidence for its origin in a benign lesion becomes progressively destroyed.

Epidemiological studies (Correa 1978) indicate that adenocarcinoma is commonest in populations in which adenomas are commonest and that within these populations the age incidence of adenomatous polyps parallel those of cancer. The peak age incidence at diagnosis of familial polyposis coli in a St Mark's Hospital series was 27.1 years, and in those patients seen in an era before prophylactic colectomy, the peak age at which carcinoma was diagnosed was 39.1 years (Morson 1974). Furthermore, in a large series of unselected patients with intestinal tumours, single adenomatous polyps of the large bowel were diagnosed at a modal age of 58.1 years, while the corresponding age at diagnosis of adenocarcinoma was 62.1 years. These data suggest that there is a long latent period during which an adenoma may be present before carcinoma develops. This latent period is probably in excess of 4 years and may even exceed 12 years.

The cardinal feature of malignancy in epithelial tumours of the large bowel is the presence of neoplastic glands infiltrating the submucosa beneath an ulcerated surface lesion. The concept of intramucosal or in situ cancer is not applicable to the large intestine. Muto et al. (1975) found foci of submucosal invasion in 46% of adenomas over 2 cm in diameter. A low incidence (1.3%) of cancer in adenomas less than 1 cm in diameter may account for the spurious impression that colorectal adenomas are not precancerous lesions.

Adenomas of large bowel also vary in their malignant potential according to their configuration. Three types are recognized (Fig. 1): tubular adenomas, tubulovillous (intermediate) adenomas, and villous adenomas (formerly called villous papillomas). Villous adenomas, frequently large, with a sea-anemone-like appearance, were found by Muto et al. (1975) to contain focal carcinoma in 40.7% of cases, whereas malignancy was only found in 4.8% of tubular adenomas and in 22.5% of intermediate lesions.

Recent Results in Cancer Research. Vol. 83

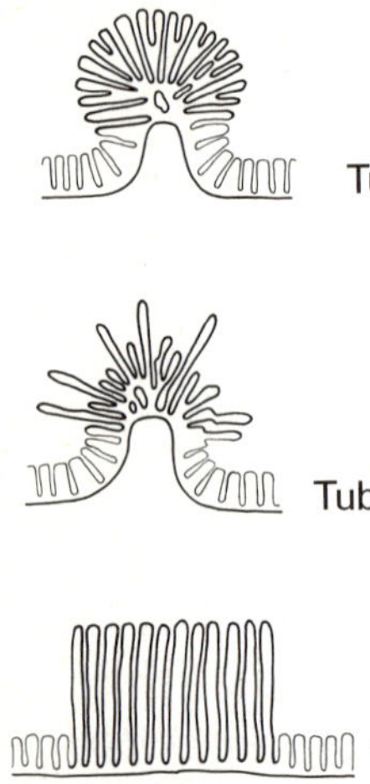

Fig. 1. Adenomas of large intestinal mucosa: variations in structure

Table 1. Five-year survival rates for adenocarcinoma of the rectum by Dukes' stage, with actuarial correction for deaths from all causes

Dukes' stage	Number	5-Year survival %
A	95	96
B	264	78
C	343	31
All cases	702	57.5

Extent of Invasion and Survival

The Dukes' classification (Dukes 1932), with good reason, is the most widely accepted way of describing the extent of local invasion by tumour at the time of operation and correlates well with survival rates (Table 1). When tumour has not infiltrated beyond the muscular coats of the large bowel (stage A) the 5-year survival rate (actuarially corrected) is comparable to that of the control population (96%).
The 5-year survival rate of patients with carcinoma infiltrating the adventitial or subserosal adipose tissue (stage B) is 78%, and when there are lymph node metastases (stage C) the 5-year survival rate falls to 31%. These figures apply to a personal series (Talbot et al. 1980) of 702 consecutive patients treated surgically for carcinoma of the rectum at St. Mark's Hospital between 1961 and 1966 with the aim of cure. It is interesting that both the proportion of patients in each Dukes' stage and the survival rates in this series are almost identical with those reported by Dukes and others nearly 50 years ago (Gabriel et al. 1935; Dukes 1957). There has thus been no improvement in the results of surgery at this specialized centre over the 50-year period. This is perhaps because there has been no change in that time in the distribution of tumour stages at the time of diagnosis (i.e., the diagnosis is not being made any earlier).

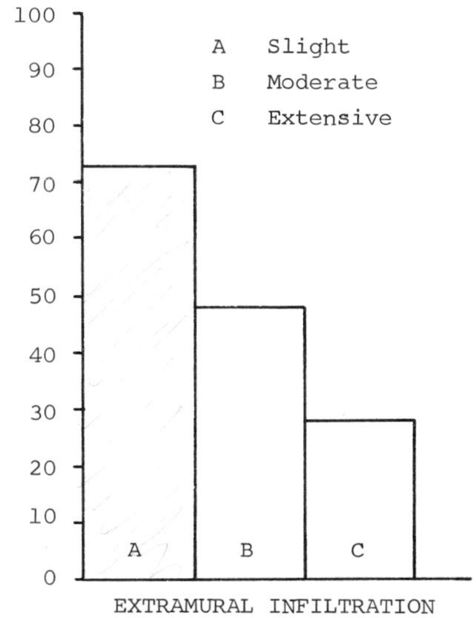

Fig. 2. Adenocarcinoma of rectum: percentage 5-year survival rates, with actuarial correction for deaths from all causes, for cases with different degrees of extramural infiltration

Table 2. Extent of extramural infiltration (numbers of cases) by Dukes' stage and actuarially corrected percentage survival rates in adenocarcinoma of the rectum

Dukes' stage	Extramural infiltration		
	Slight	Moderate	Extensive
B	(141) 73%	(66) 61%	(55) 45%
C	(85) 43%	(95) 25%	(144) 15%

Amongst the tumours of Dukes' stage B or C there are some which only infiltrate slightly into the perirectal adipose tissue ('early' B/C cases), while others extensively infiltrate the subserosa or adventitia, sometimes involving the peritoneum or even adjacent organs such as the prostate, uterus, or vagina. Other tumours show an intermediate extent of extramural infiltration somewhere between the above two extremes. There is a direct relationship between the corrected 5-year survival rate and the extent of extramural invasion at the time of operation (Fig. 2). However, extent of invasion does not outweigh the influence on prognosis of the presence of lymph node metastases, as can be seen from Table 2. This shows how the 5-year survival rates vary according to extent of extramural tumour infiltration for both Dukes' stage B and C cases. The classic Dukes' staging procedure remains the most effective way of classifying colorectal cancer for prognostic purposes, despite recent alternative suggestions (Wood 1980).

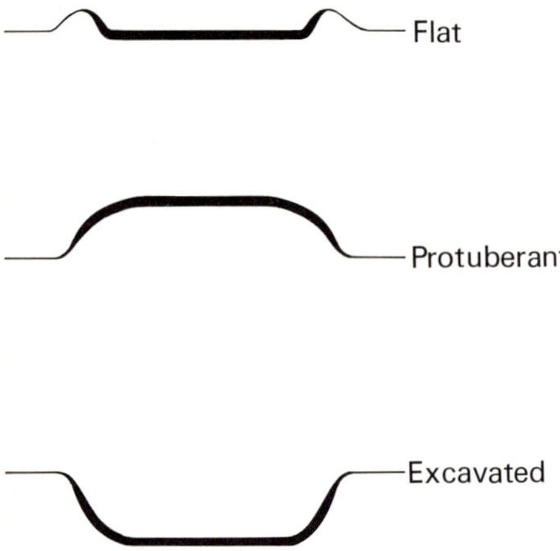

Fig. 3. Adenocarcinoma of rectum: three types of tumour configuration

Table 3. Configurations of growth in adenocarcinoma, with numbers of patients surviving operation, and corrected 5-year survival rates

Configuration	Number	5-Year survival %
Protuberant	157	70
Flat	469	58
Excavated	58	16

Gross Morphology and Prognosis

The gross morphology of colorectal carcinomas is typically flat and ulcerated with slightly raised edges (Fig. 3) but sometimes there is a protuberant polyp-like mass. Alternatively there may be a large, deeply excavated crater. Over two-thirds of 684 consecutive rectal carcinomas examined at St Mark's Hospital were flat (Table 3), less than 25% were protuberant, and approximately one in twelve tumours was excavated. The corrected 5-year survival rate was high for patients with protuberant tumours (70%), low (16%) when the tumours were excavated, and intermediate (58%) for flat tumours.

One of the properties of colorectal cancer is that it infiltrates directly out through the bowel wall and, in contrast to gastric cancer, malignant cells do not infiltrate sideways beneath an intact mucosa. Measurement of the diameter of a mucosal lesion therefore gives a good indication of the total size of the mass. It may be supposed that the diameter of a tumour could provide an alternative parameter to the Dukes' stage which would allow a *pre-operative* prognostic assessment. As Fig. 4 shows, there is indeed a relatively good (70%) survival rate in cases with a tumour diameter of less than 2 cm. However, there is no significant relationship between survival rate and size of tumours over 2 cm. One reason for this may be that some tumours appear spuriously large because they are complicated by an inflammatory reaction or even abscess formation. Since most colorectal cancers are at least 4 cm in diameter at diagnosis there is little hope that tumour size can be useful for assessing prognosis.

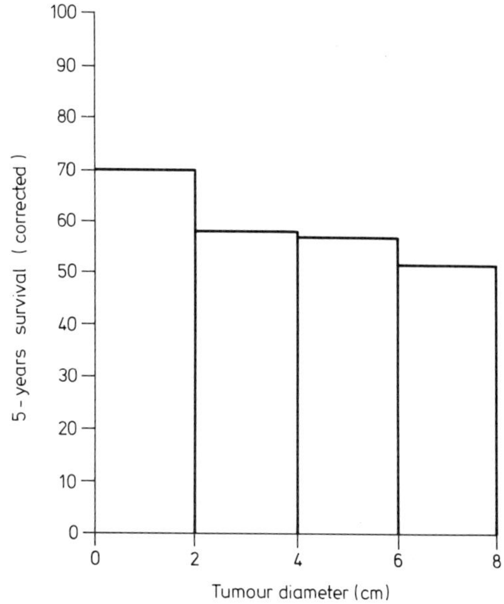

Fig. 4. Adenocarcinoma of rectum: percentage 5-year survival rates, with actuarial correction for cases with different tumour sizes

Cause of Death and Pattern of Tumour Dissemination

All surviving patients in this personal series were carefully followed up for at least 5 years and accurate records kept of the pattern of tumour spread at the time of death (Table 4). Two hundred and ninety-seven (42%) of the 703 patients died as a result of recurrent tumour, either local or distant. Of all patients in the series, 25% developed liver metastases. The next most frequent secondary site at death was the lung (10%). Local pelvic recurrence was present in 8.5% of patients and metastases at other sites such as bone, peritoneum, brain, adrenal, and kidney developed in 3% of patients or less.

Pathogenesis of Distant Metastases: Venous Invasion

It is self-evident that before a metastatic tumour can develop in distant sites such as liver, lung, brain, and bone, carcinoma cells must embolize through the bloodstream (Willis 1973). It remains uncertain how and where the tumour cells enter the bloodstream. The traditional view has followed the concept of Stiles (1899) that initially carcinoma cells spread via lymphatics and that spread via the bloodstream follows from this. However, histological evidence of invasion of rectal veins by adenocarcinoma has been demonstrated in 52% of the cases in one study (Talbot et al. 1980).

Distant metastases often develop when no lymph node deposits are found. That invasion of veins is directly related to blood-borne dissemination is suggested by the difference in survival rates between patients with and without spread of this kind which has been demonstrated by Talbot (1980). In patients in whom venous invasion was observed the corrected 5-year survival rate was significantly lower (43%) than when venous spread was not demonstrated (73%).

Table 4. Pattern of tumour spread in patients dying with adenocarcinoma of the rectum (i.e., 'recurrence')

Deaths from recurrence	297	(42%)
Liver metastases	176	(25%)
Lung metastases	69	(10%)
Local pelvic recurrence	60	(8.5%)
Bone metastases	22	(3%)
Peritoneal spread	18	(3%)
Brain metastases	18	(3%)
Other metastases	15	(2%)

Table 5. Configuration of growth in adenocarcinoma of the rectum, with total numbers of cases and incidence of venous invasion

Configuration of growth	Number	Venous invasion observed %
Protuberant	163	36
Flat	479	55
Excavated	61	70

That venous invasion is an inherent property of rectal carcinoma and is related to tumour invasiveness is suggested by a study of the relationship between the incidence of venous invasion and the gross configuration of tumour (Table 5). Venous spread was observed in only 36% of protuberant growths, whereas there was evidence of invasion of veins in 70% of excavated tumours, flat growths falling mid-way between the two extremes. If one regards excavated tumours as the most aggressive and protuberant growths as the least invasive the significance of vein invasion is evident.

Invasion of veins by rectal cancer follows a histological pattern which is described in detail elsewhere (Talbot et al. 1981). There appears to be an inflammatory reaction in the host tissues to the presence of necrotic tumour within veins. This results in damage to the vein walls and the formation of a protective cap of endothelium covering the permeating growth as part of a process of endophlebitis obliterans. Malignant embolism is thus inhibited, whereas when is only a slight chronic inflammatory reaction in and around the vein wall blood-borne metastasis is more likely.

Embolisms & blood borne metastasis.

Venous Invasion, Dukes' Stage, and Survival

The combination of venous invasion and local invasion as measured by the Dukes' stage has an additive effect on survival (Fig. 5). The observation of invasion of veins (intramural only) in stage A cases is not related to survival but when extramural venous invasion is observed in stage B and C cases there is a significant worsening of survival rates. This is particularly so when thick-walled extramural veins are involved.

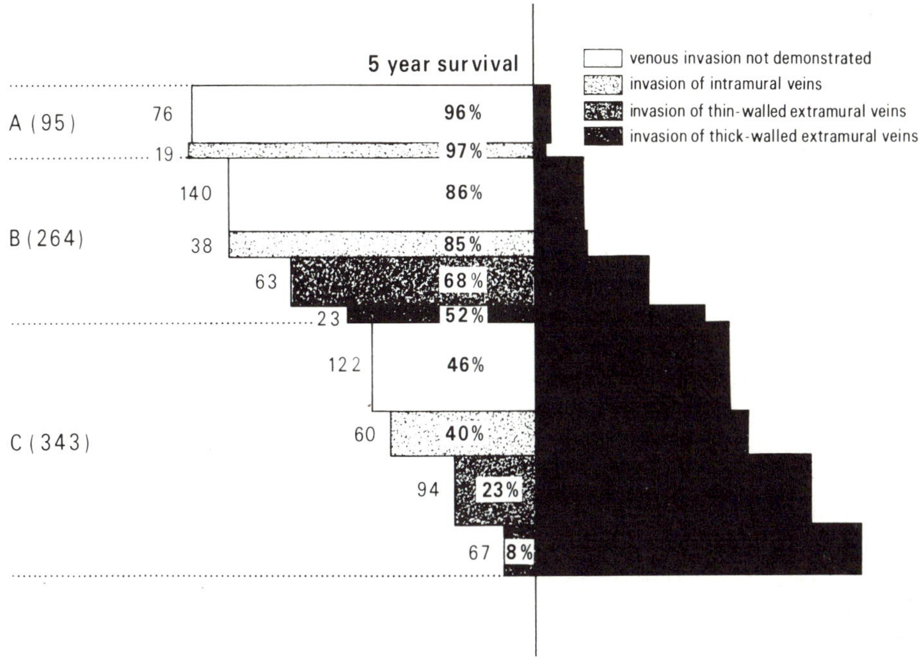

Fig. 5. Adenocarcinoma of rectum: actuarial correction of 5-year survival rates, Dukes' stage, and venous invasion of primary growth. Total numbers of each group are shown on the *left*, mortality rates in black on the *right*

The corrected 5-year survival rate for patients with stage C tumours when there is spread into thick-walled extramural veins is only 8.5%.

Conclusions

The surgical treatment of colorectal cancer now appears to have reached a plateau of success. Prevention of the disease by detection and removal of precancerous lesions, particularly adenomatous polyps, has never been more urgently needed. The staging procedure originally proposed by Dukes remains a most useful method of assessing prognosis. The survival rate of patients is also directly proportional to the extent of extramural invasion by tumour at the time of operation. Patients with tumours under 2 cm in diameter and with protuberant tumours have a relatively better chance of survival. Patients with large and excavated tumours have a poor prognosis. Forty-two percent of patients are likely to die as a result of local or distant recurrent tumour, and 25% of patients are likely to develop liver metastases.

Invasion of extramural veins correlates with the extent of local invasion and is associated with the development of liver and other distant metastases. There is some variation in host reaction in venous invasion which may influence malignant embolism.

Any radical improvement in mortality from colorectal cancer is likely to come from prevention, by excision of the premalignant lesion, or from *earlier diagnosis, before extramural venous invasion is established,* with its inherent tendency to blood-borne metastasis. Radiology may have a part to play here, as improved techniques allow detection of increasingly small lesions.

Future management of the established disease is likely to involve new modes of treatment, such as adjuvant radiotherapy and chemotherapy. The increased precision of prognostic prediction which results from combining the Dukes' staging with an assessment of venous invasion should provide a firm base upon which to evaluate the relative effectiveness of new forms of therapy. It should also make it possible to select those patients with particularly aggressive tumours who are most likely to benefit from adjuvant therapy.

References

Correa P (1978) Epidemiology of polyps and cancer. In: Morson BC (ed) The pathogenesis of colorectal cancer. Saunders, London, pp 126–152

Day DW, Morson BC (1978) The adenoma-carcinoma sequence. In: Morson BC (ed) The pathogenesis of colorectal cancer. Saunders, London, pp 58–71

Dukes CE (1932) The classification of cancer of the rectum. J Pathol Bacteriol 35: 1489–1494

Dukes CE (1957) Discussion on major surgery in carcinoma of the rectum with or without colostomy, excluding the anal canal and including the rectosigmoid. Proc R Soc Med 50: 1031–1052

Gabriel WB, Dukes CE, Bussey HJR (1935) Lymphatic spread in cancer of the rectum. Br J Surg 23: 395–413

Horn RC (1971) Malignant potential of polypoid lesions of the colon and rectum. Cancer 28: 146–152

Morson BC (1974) The polyp-cancer sequence in the large bowel. Proc R Soc Med 67: 451–457

Muto T, Bussey HJR, Morson BC (1975) The evolution of cancer of the colon and rectum. Cancer 36: 2251–2270

Riddel RH, Shove DC, Ritchie JK, Lennard-Jones JE, Morson BC (1978) Precancer in ulcerative colitis. In: Morson BC (ed) The pathogenesis of colorectal cancer. Saunders, London, pp 95–118

Stiles HJ (1899) On the dissemination of cancer of the breast. Br Med J 1: 1452–1459

Talbot IC (1980) Spread of rectal cancer within veins and mechanisms of malignant embolism. In: Wright R (ed) Recent advances in gastrointestinal pathology. Saunders, London, pp 353–364

Talbot IC, Ritchie S, Leighton MH, Hughes AO, Bussey HJR, Morson BC (1980) The clinical significance of invasion of veins by rectal cancer. Br J Surg 67: 439–442

Talbot IC, Ritchie S, Leighton M, Hughes AO, Bussey HJR, Morson BC (1981) Invasion of veins by carcinoma of rectum: method of detection, histological features and significance. Histopathology 5: 141–163

Willis R (1973) The spread of tumours in the human body, 3rd edn. Butterworths, London, pp 37–42

Wood CB (1980) Prognostic factors in staging of colorectal cancer. In: Welvaart K, Blumgart LH, Kreuning J (eds) Colorectal cancer. Leiden University Press, The Hague Boston London, pp 29–42

Biochemical Markers

E. H. Cooper and J. O'Quigley

Unit for Cancer Research, University of Leeds, Leeds LS2 9NL, United Kingdom

Biochemical changes in colorectal cancer vary considerably according to the stage, the disease, and the tumour burden. The search for tumour markers in this disease has been of considerable interest since the early descriptions of carcinoembryonic antigen by Gold and Freedman (1965) and the realization that CEA levels in the plasma could be used to monitor the evolution of certain forms of gastrointestinal cancer (Hansen et al. 1974; Moore et al. 1971; MacKay et al. 1974). Since this pioneer work, CEA has been the subject of many reviews. One of the more recent, by Ladenson and McDonald (1980), provides a guide to the main literature on this topic. To rehearse this information yet again is probably unhelpful. Instead we have chosen to report and discuss the experience gained in Leeds in the monitoring of large-bowel cancer from 1974 to 1981 and try to identify some of the reasons why it is still difficult to make many definitive statements about biochemical monitoring and the advantages and limitations of the systems currently available.

Materials and Methods

The patients were initially drawn from the Department of Surgery (Prof. J. C. Goligher), where the treatment policy was surgery for the primary lesion and symptomatic treatment for recurrence, but chemotherapy was not employed. Later, patients studied by members of the Yorkshire Gastrointestinal Cancer Research Group (Chairman: Prof. G. R. Giles) were examined. Their policy was to use various chemotherapy protocols as a second-line treatment following surgical resection of the primary tumour. In the main, chemotherapy was used in advanced disease with indicator lesions. Some protocols were for the treatment of patients with minimal residual disease or with a high risk of recurrence (Dukes' C) (Lawton et al. 1980).

Two forms of CEA assay were used. In the earlier part of our studies the double-antibody assay described by Laurence et al. (1972) and run at the Chester Beatty Institute (Prof. M. Neville) was used. This assay had an upper limit of normal of 30 ng/ml. More recently we have evaluated the Abbott CEA-EIA assay, with an upper limit of normal of 5 ng/ml. Gamma-glutamyl transpeptidase (γGT) was estimated by the method of Jacobs (1971), while albumin (ALB), pre-albumin (P-ALB), C-reactive protein (C-RP), and transferrin (TSF) were measured immunochemically by single radial immunodiffusion with specific antisera.

The statistical approach to this investigation is outlined in Appendix 1.

Results of Pre- and Postoperative Assessment

An assessment has been made of the contribution of pre-operative measurements of CEA, γGT, and CEA (Laurence assay) and the change of these measurements that occurs 2–3 months after surgery, and of the patients' survival. The 145 patients studied in this series were all treated by Professor Goligher and staged according to a strict protocol. The ages ranged between 28 and 86 years, with a median age of 66 years. There were 79 males and 66 females. Dukes' A or B lesions accounted for 49% of the sample (71 patients), Dukes' C lesions, 32% of the sample (47 patients), and metastatic disease at the time of surgery (stage D), 19% of the sample (27 patients).

A multivariate statistical model made it possible to perform a sequential investigation of the factors influencing survival (Appendix 1). Factors are entered into the model in a stepwise manner. The criterion for inclusion in the model is the addition of prognostic information to that already known, and this is described in Appendix 1. The results of this approach are illustrated in Table 1.

The most important factor to be included in the model was Dukes' stage, as may have been expected. However, within a given Dukes' stage, survival varied considerably according to pre-operative CEA and γGT levels and according to the extent to which they changed after surgery. The stepwise technique allowed us to conclude that pre-operative CEA levels carried prognostic information supplementary to the Dukes' stage. At this point the level of γGT measured pre-operatively seemed to carry no helpful information. However, the change in γGT over the course of 2 months not only contributed significantly itself to explaining survival, but once included in the model enabled the initial pre-operative γGT measurement also to be included. At first glance this result seems paradoxical, but in fact it lends itself to a simple interpretation. In itself the initial γGT is not informative, but when combined with the knowledge of how it changes after operation it becomes important. Thus if there is a drop in γGT levels but the initial level was high this is less important than a drop at a lower level. These pieces of biochemical information, although they may be highly significant statistically, are not necessarily of great clinical importance individually. Thus the survival of patients, as predicted by a lower (18.2 ng/ml), an average (28.0 ng/ml), and a high level (41 ng/ml) of pre-operative CEA, does not differ greatly (Fig. 1). The CEA level is evidently of much less prognostic value than Dukes' stage (Fig. 2). If, however, as has been indicated by the model, these biochemical measurements can

Table 1. Stepwise inclusion of terms

Term[a]	χ^2 (−2 log [likelihood ratio])	p
Dukes' stage	32.2	< 0.001
Dukes' stage, CEA	22.6	< 0.001
Dukes' stage, γGT	3.5	NS
Dukes' stage, CEA, $\Delta\gamma$GT	6.2	< 0.02
Dukes' stage, CEA, $\Delta\gamma$GT, γGT	8.0	< 0.005
Dukes' stage, CEA, $\Delta\gamma$GT, γGT, ΔCEA	4.5	< 0.05

[a] $\Delta\gamma$GT, change between pre-operative γGT and 2-month postoperative level; ΔCEA, change between pre-operative CEA and 2-month postoperative level

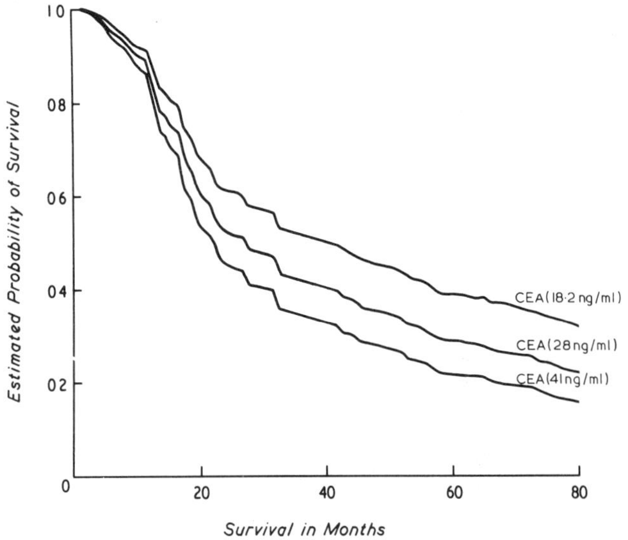

Fig. 1. Survival according to pre-operative CEA levels. (1) 18.2 ng/ml, (2) 28.0 ng/ml, (3) 41.0 ng/ml. Estimated Cox's model

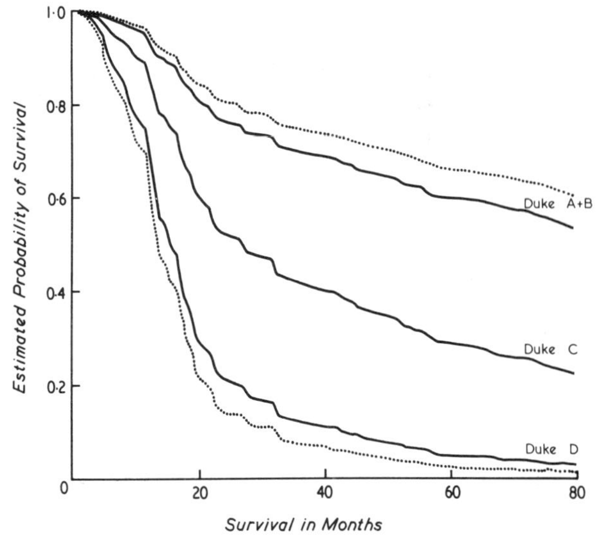

Fig. 2. Survival according to stage. *Heavy lines* refer to Dukes' stage. *Dotted lines* show the survival probability estimates for the two Dukes' C cases described in the text

contribute independent pieces of prognostic information then adding them all together provides a powerful index. Thus a consideration of the pre-operative levels of CEA and γGT and the differences between these pre-operative levels and those taken 2 months later can help identify patients with very different prognostic outlooks. These differences exist within the potentially curative stages A, B, and C as well as within stage D.

Figure 2 contrasts the estimated survival probabilities (Appendix 1) between different Dukes' stages for this data set and they agree closely with those of much larger series (Moertel 1973). The two dotted lines represent estimated survival probabilities for a patient with a Dukes' C lesion but differing CEA and γGT levels. If the patient initially had high pre-operative serum levels (CEA 41 ng/ml, γGT 42 U/l) and 2 months after the operation these levels had increased, on the basis of our experience the calculated survival probabilities can be seen to be even poorer than for stage D as a whole. In striking contrast, if the initial levels were lower (CEA 19 ng/ml, γGT 19 U/l) and following the operation they decreased then the estimated survival probabilities are better than the expected overall survival rates for the combined group of patients with Dukes' stage A and B cancers. It is clear, then, that these methods go some way to explaining the observed variability in survival within any given Dukes' stage. Potential applications of these findings are considered in the discussion.

Postoperative Monitoring of Minimal Residual Disease

The probability of recurrence is well-recognized to be associated with the Dukes' stage as crude 5-year survival rates are 61%–81% for stage A, 25%–64% for stage B, and 6%–28% for stage C according to four major studies (Moertel et al. 1973). However, although some refinement of the broad prognostic indices is possible, the earliest warning of occult recurrence or metastases still appears to be a rising CEA. The lead time given by this test depends on the frequency of the measurement of the levels. In a closely monitored group of patients who remained tumour-free after resection, it was found that the variation of CEA was small about each individual's own mean, but levels of < 1–6 ng CEA-EIA/ml were all compatible with health (Table 2). The rates of rise of CEA and the duration of time with normal values prior to the rise vary considerably (Fig. 3). However, experience suggests that testing every 3 months will provide the optimum, and an economic, schedule if the surgeon or oncologist wishes to know whether the CEA is rising and whether the probability of a recurrence or metastasis has greatly increased in these patients. Such testing will not indicate the site of the disease, and in our experience neither will γGT as it is not sensitive to small volumes of hepatic metastases (Cooper and Munro Neville 1978). In the more aggressive tumours rapidly rising CEA and γGT levels usually indicate extensive hepatic metastases. It must be borne in mind that occasional spurious rises of CEA can occur, which may reflect a temporary alteration in production or degradation. In our experience, coincidental chronic benign liver disease is an uncommon event.

Table 2. CEA levels in tumour-free patients after resection of primary large bowel cancer

Patient	Follow-up in months	No. of observations	CEA-EIA Mean ng/ml	SD
E.T.	39	15	1.74	0.29
M.A.	17	6	1.5	0.39
E.N.	23	13	5.49	0.52
C.E.	25	12	2.25	0.31
S.L.	28	15	1.74	1.90
E.S.[a]	19	12	1.08	0.27
C.S.[a]	11	11	1.65	1.06
M.D.[a]	23	10	3.85	1.22

[a] Adjuvant therapy

In the monitoring of patients receiving chemotherapy for minimal residual disease, Lawton et al. (1980) reported an experience of 43 patients with known residual disease of small tumour bulk that could not be detected after resection; the rates of rise of the CEA (Laurence assay) were of interest. In the fast-rising pattern the levels reached 100 ng/ml or higher at 6 months in an intermediate pattern they reached; 30–100 ng/ml, and in one group CEA levels did not rise. Nine of ten patients in the first group showed progression within 12 months, and seven had died. At 1 year, only 5 of the 25 who showed no rise had evidence of progression, whilst 5 out of the 7 with an intermediate rise showed evidence of progression (2 of these patients died). In this study it was apparent that chemotherapy slowed the rise of CEA, and a rapidly rising CEA whilst the patient was receiving chemotherapy was a strong indication that such treatment was having no beneficial effect.

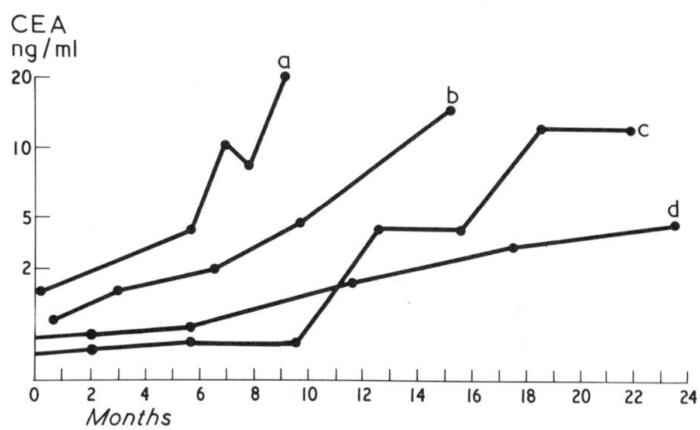

Fig. 3. Slow rates of rise of serum CEA (Abbott EIA) in patients with recurrent or metastatic colorectal cancer; patients c and d had antecedent values of < 2 ng/ml for 15 and 12 months, respectively

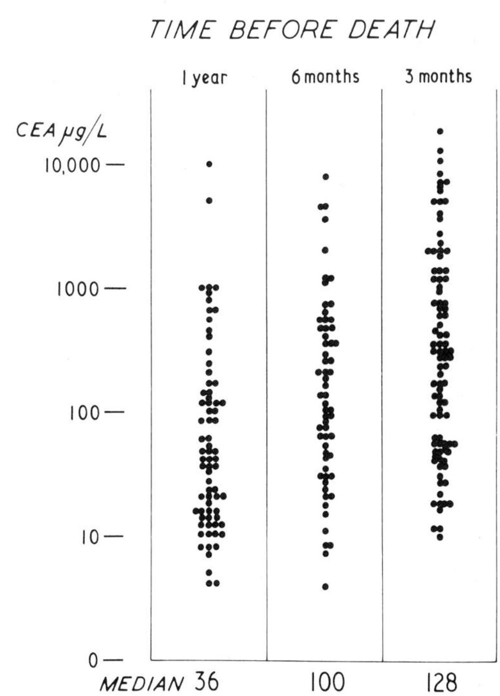

Fig. 4. Distribution of serum CEA (Laurence assay) in patients with incurable metastatic or recurrent colorectal cancer. [From Milano et al. (1978) J Nat Cancer Inst]

Monitoring of Advanced Cancer

Earlier experience showed that levels of CEA in advanced colorectal cancer can vary greatly, as is shown in Fig. 4. It will be seen that the median level rises as the patients approach death, but the variability remains very large. About 10%–20% show no evidence of a raised CEA at any time in the illness even when death is the result of carcinomatosis.

A reappraisal of this information came from patients being treated for advanced colorectal cancer; this time the Abbott CEA-EIA assay was used. In 24 patients, who were first seen with an initial CEA level that was raised (> 5 ng/ml) but still less than 20 ng/ml the median survival was 7 months from first attendance at the clinic, whilst in 37 with an initial CEA > 20 ng/ml the median survival was 4 months. However, the ranges of survival times in the two groups were 3–36 months and 0.5–32 months, respectively. Thirty-two percent of these 61 patients had an initial CEA of > 100 ng/ml.

Carcinoembryonic Antigen

A comparison of a monoclonal CEA assay (MA/1) and two routine assays, Abbott EIA and the Charing Cross assay, has been made in longitudinal studies of 33 patients with colorectal cancer (Rogers et al. 1981). This demonstrated the MA/1 did not increase the prognostic reliability by adding a monoclonal to a routine CEA. However, it was apparent that colorectal tumours express different forms of CEA, which are recognized differently by each of the three assays. The future use of monoclonal assays will depend on finding particular CEA antibodies that can provide information useful to clinicians. Such assays have the advantage of being more closely defined than the polyvalent systems.

Non-Specific Changes in Plasma Proteins

Patients with advanced cancer exhibit a variety of non-specific changes in plasma protein levels. The tendency is for those proteins that reflect the nutritional status to fall, and the acute phase reactant proteins (APRPs) to rise. Both are integrated cascades that show an overall correlation but considerable variability from one patient to another for the same apparent tumour burden. To examine this phenomenon it is convenient to synchronize the data with respect to the patients' death and then work backwards from this point.

Each patient contributes a series of data points corresponding to protein measurements at different times. A visual inspection is sufficient to indicate an overall fall in the nutritional proteins and a tendency for the APRPs to precede this fall by increasing their serum concentration. It has been suggested that the statistical methods of time series analysis may be helpful in resolving similar problems. In this context, however, that has not been the case. The paucity of measurements in each individual and the fact that intervals between measurements are almost inevitably unequal means that the time series analysis techniques are inappropriate. Regression models used in survival analysis are also inappropriate, as they rely upon maximum likelihood techniques which assume independence between successive observations. However, simpler methods which estimate the rates of change of protein levels are sufficient to highlight the phenomena of interest.

The rise of APRPs seen in most patients is illustrated by reference to C-reactive protein. In patients with advanced colorectal cancer 6–12 months prior to death 69% had normal levels, 16% a moderate increase, and 16% a marked increase. During the last 3 months of life only 10% had normal levels, and a marked increase (> 50 mg/litre) was present in 63% (Cooper and Turner 1980).

There is a strong correlation between APRPs, so that similar information can be obtained from measurement of orosomucoid (α_1-acid glycoprotein) or antichymotrypsin; the phenotypic variation of α_1-antitrypsin and haptoglobin make them less suitable as indicators. The interdependence of these systems is illustrated in Fig. 5, which shows how pre-albumin levels (PALB) and retinol-binding protein (RBP), indicators of nutrition, are much lower when APRPs are raised. Occasionally, unexpected high RBP levels will occur when the PALB is low; this is normally due to an excess of the free form of RBP, which is a low molecular weight protein and dependent on the kidney for its clearance from the blood. In these patients, a raised serum creatinine and reduced glomerular filtration rate will usually account for the discrepancy.

The rates of change of the plasma protein concentrations and the order in which abnormalities occur in the cascade varies. During the last 3 months of life the most rapid and severe changes will occur but will not necessarily be accompanied by any further weight loss as shown in Fig. 6.

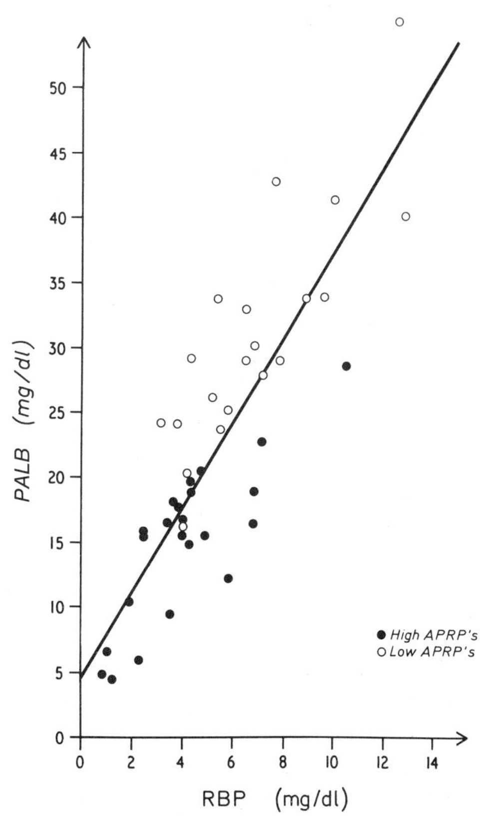

Fig. 5. Relationship of serum prealbumin and retinol-binding protein concentration and the levels of acute phase reactant proteins in bladder cancer

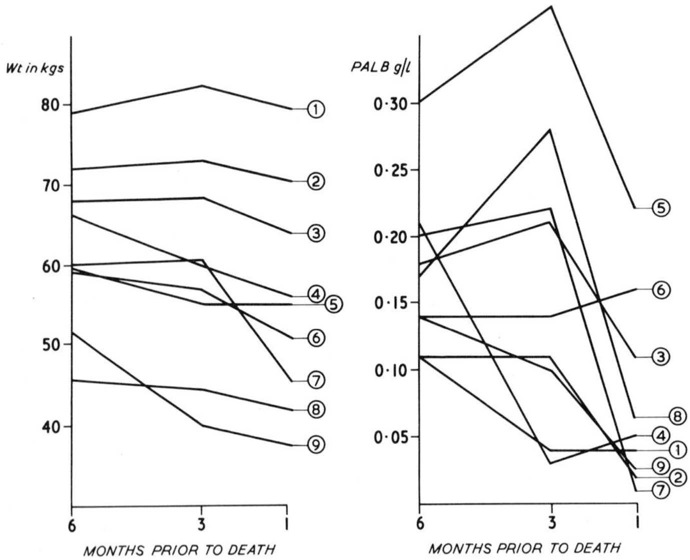

Fig. 6. Fall in weight of patients with advanced colorectal cancer compared with the fall of prealbumin concentration. [From Milano et al. (1978) J Natl Cancer Inst]

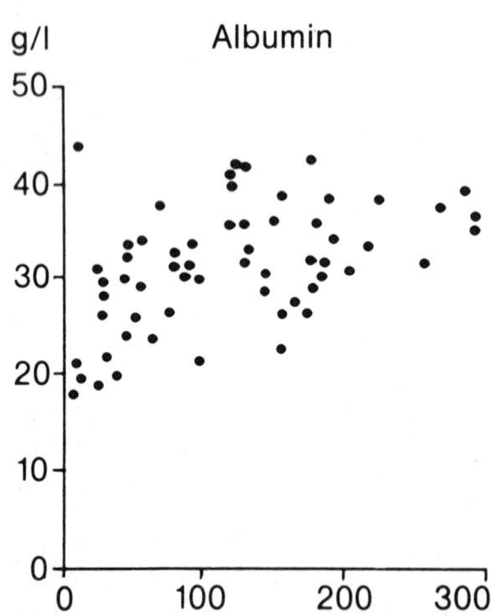

Fig. 7. Levels of serum albumin at various times prior to death in patients with colorectal cancer

Serum albumin, having a far larger pool size than the APRPs or PALB, tends to level out the minor oscillation of levels seen in these other proteins, but a terminal fall is usual (Fig. 7). The rate of fall of albumin can be a long slow decline or may be accentuated in the preterminal state depending on the metabolic effects of the tumour and its mass (Hall 1979).

Application in the Analysis of Clinical Trials

In clinical trials a stratification based upon Dukes' stage is usually employed to ensure prognostic comparability between different treatment groups. It is clear, however, that within each stage, and in particular after potentially curative therapy, the wide variability in survival rates may often conceal an improvement in treatment. This will be particularly so in trials with small numbers where a high probability may exist of the randomization producing treatment groups with significantly different prognostic features.

A careful assessment of certain biochemical variants, however, considerably refines prognostic determinations and can therefore improve the sensitivity of any trial. Modern methods of statistical analysis do not require a randomization on the basis of these factors. Providing they are measured for each entrant to a trial, appropriate statistical adjustments can be made at the time of analysis. It is probable that a similar approach could be used for patients with advanced colorectal cancer and an indicator lesion entered into phase II trials. In these circumstances longitudinal measurements would be essential.

Appendix 1. Statistical Evaluation

From a statistical viewpoint postoperative survival time, t, may be regarded as a random variable. The probability that a patient will survive beyond any given time t is a function of t, known as the survivorship function S(t). It is necessary to investigate how this function is related to other variables $X_1, X_2 \ldots X_p$. A useful approach employs the hazard function, h(t), which is related directly to S(t). Roughly speaking, the hazard is proportional to the probability of failing in a small time interval, given that the patient has at least survived until the beginning of the interval. Cox (1972) defines a regression model in which the hazard is related to the other variables $X_1, X_2 \ldots X_p$ by

$$h(t) = h_0(t) \exp(\Sigma_j \beta_j X_j) \quad (1)$$

where $h_0(t)$ is unknown and remains unspecified. A technique analogous to that of maximum likelihood (Cox 1975) is used to estimate the βs when $h_0(t)$ is not known. These techniques permit likelihood ratio tests on subsets of parameters to be made in the same way as with ordinary maximum likelihood. Thus we can compare a model in which certain of the βs are fixed at zero against on where they are allowed to vary. If the latter model provides a better fit to the former, as indicated by sufficiently large values of $-2 \log$ (likelihood ratio), when compared with χ^2 tables, then this is regarded as evidence that those terms corresponding to the non-zero coefficients influence survival.

Once the βs have been estimated $h_0(t)$ and therefore $S_0(t)$ can themselves be estimated from the data. There are a number of approaches to this and we use one suggested by Breslow (1974). A survivorship function, $S(t; X_1 \ldots X_p)$, corresponding to a patient with non-zero $X_1, \ldots X_p$ follows directly from Eq. (1) and is given by

$$S(t; X_1 \ldots X_p) = [S_0(t)] \exp(\Sigma_j \beta_j X_j) \,. \quad (2)$$

Thus, if any values of the X_i are known for a particular patient it is possible to calculate a survivorship function, and hence probabilities associated with survival beyond given times. How meaningful such probabilities are in reality depends upon how well the regression model describes the situation. As with ordinary regression, caution is required when extrapolating beyond the immediate range of validity, and of course if the linear multiplicative model is too severe an approximation then estimated probabilities may be quite different from actual ones. Nonetheless, if we only include in the model terms shown to influence survival strongly, as indicated by high levels of significance, then the calculated probabilities relative to each other provide a helpful guide to the identification of different prognostic groupings.

References

Breslow NE (1974) Covariance analysis of censored survival data. Biometrics 30: 89–99

Cooper EH, Munro Neville A (1978) Logic and logistics of monitoring large bowel cancer. In: Lipkin M, Good RA (eds) Gastrointestinal tract cancer. Plenum Press, New York, pp 437–455

Cooper EH, Turner R (1980) Multiparametric approach to biochemical surveillance of large-bowel cancer. In: Winawer S, Schottenfeld D, Sherlock P (eds) Colorectal cancer: Prevention, epidemiology and screening. Raven Press, New York, pp 211–218

Cox DR (1972) Regression models and life tables (with discussion). J R Statist Soc [B] 34: 187–220

Cos DR (1975) Partial likelihood. Biometrika 62: 269–276

Gold P, Freedman S (1965) Demonstration of tumourspecific antigens in human colonic carcinomata by immunological tolerance and absorption techniques. J Exp Med 121: 439–462

Hall JC (1979) The cachexia of cancer. Biomedicine 30: 287–290

Hansen HJ, Snyder JJ, Miller E, Vandevoorde JP, Miller ON, Hines LR, Burns JJ (1974) Carcinoembryonic antigen (CEA) assay: a laboratory adjunct in the diagnosis and management of cancer. J Hum Pathol 5: 139–147

Jacobs WLW (1971) Colorimetric assay for γ-glutamyl transpeptidase. Clin Chim Acta 31: 175–179

Ladenson JH, McDonald JM (1980) Colorectal carcinoma and carcinoembryonic antigen (CEA). Clin Chem 26: 1213–1220

Laurence DJR, Stevens U, Dettelhiem R, Darcy C, Leese C, Tuberville C, Alexander P, Jones EW, Neville AM (1972) Role of plasma carcinoembryonic antigen in diagnosis of gastrointestinal, mammary and bronchial carcinoma. Br Med J 3: 605–609

Lawton JO, Giles GR, Cooper EH (1980) Evaluation of CEA in patients with known residual disease after resection of colonic cancer. J R Soc Med 73: 23–28

MacKay AM, Patel S, Carter S, Stevens U, Laurence DJR, Cooper EH, Neville AM (1974) Role of serial CEA assays in detection of recurrent and metastatic colorectal carcinomas. Br Med J 4: 382–385

Milano G, Cooper EH, Goligher JC, Giles GR, Neville AM (1978) Serum prealbumin, retinol-binding protein, transferrin and albumin levels in patients with large-bowel cancer. J Natl Cancer Inst 61: 687–691

Moertel C (1973) Large bowel. In: Holland JF, Frei E (eds) Cancer medicine. Lea & Febiger, Philadelphia, pp 1597–1626

Moore TL, Kupchik HZ, Marcon N (1971) Carcinoembryonic antigen assays in cancer of the colon and pancreas and other digestive tract disorders. Am J Digest Dis 16: 1–7

Rogers GT, Rawlins GA, Bagshawe KD (1981) Somatic-cell hybrids producing antibodies against CEA. Br J Cancer 43: 1–4

Radiological Assessment

D. J. Nolan

Department of Diagnostic Radiology, John Radcliffe Hospital,
Oxford OX3 9DM, United Kingdom

A complete radiological assessment is important for the proper diagnosis and management of cancer of the colon and rectum. Plain abdominal radiographs should be the initial investigation in patients who present with symptoms or signs of intestinal obstruction. Radionuclide studies, ultrasound, and computerized tomography are now available and can be used for detecting the presence of hepatic metastases. The barium examination of the colon remains one of the most important diagnostic procedures and when properly performed is accurate in detecting primary cancers of the colon that are beyond the reach of the sigmoidoscope. However, if the barium enema examination is poorly performed lesions will be missed and the clinician will be led to believe that the colon is normal. The resulting delay in diagnosis can mean that there is further spread of the primary tumour and the opportunity for early diagnosis with a good prognosis will be missed. When the cancer has spread into the bowel wall, but not beyond the muscularis propria, and there are no lymph node metastases (Dukes' A) the patient is almost invariably cured of his disease by appropriate surgical treatment (Morson and Dawson 1979). If the growth has spread beyond the muscularis propria into the pericolic or perirectal tissues in continuity, but there are no regional lymph node metastases (Dukes' B), there is a 70% chance of being cured. When the lymph nodes are involved (Dukes' C) the prognosis is poor, with only about a 1 in 3 chance of the patient surviving 5 years.

There is evidence that cancers of the colon arise from previously benign adenomas (Muto et al. 1975). The barium enema examination should therefore be sensitive enough to detect small polyps of the colon as well as cancers. Most radiologists now agree that the double-contrast barium enema should be used routinely for detecting cancers and polyps of the colon. A clean colon, suitable barium suspension, air insufflation, and the routine use of smooth muscle relaxant drugs together with a good radiographic technique are essential for consistently good results. Cancers of the colon may be missed because of poor preparation, faulty technique, or inadequate attention to detail (Miller 1976).

A double-contrast barium enema is contraindicated if there is suspected perforation of the colon or toxic megacolon. If obstruction or complications of diverticular disease, such as localized abscess or fistula formation, are suspected, a single-contrast barium enema should be performed. The single-contrast enema can sometimes be helpful in confirming the presence of a carcinoma of the caecum or ascending colon if there has been poor mucosal coating of that area on the double-contrast examination. Excellent visualization of the caecum and ascending colon as well as the distal ileum can be obtained by administering barium orally and introducting air rectally when the barium is in the region of the caecum (Kellett et al. 1977). The patient is prepared as for a

Recent Results in Cancer Research. Vol. 83

double-contrast enema and then barium suspension is taken orally. The progress of the barium column is checked and when the head of the column reaches the transverse colon, air is introduced rectally and radiographs are taken. Carcinoma of the caecum and Crohn's disease are particularly well demonstrated by this technique.

Double-Contrast Barium Enema

Colon Preparation

The barium enema is probably the most neglected and poorly performed examination in the field of radiology (Miller 1976). Eighteen percent, or more, of cancers of the colon are missed on the initial barium enema examination (Saunders and MacEwen 1971). In most cases the cancer is missed because it is obscured or mistaken for faecal material. A clean colon is therefore the most important part of the barium enema examination. Complete responsibility for obtaining a clean colon must be assumed by the radiologist (Miller 1975). A combination of diet, increased fluid intake, laxatives, and a cleansing enema are essential for consistently getting the colon clean. The examination is best performed on an out-patient basis whenever possible. Clear instructions should be given to the patient, pointing out the importance of a clean colon and the rigorous preparation required. The method described by Miller (1975) gives consistently good results.

Diet

The patient is restricted to a low-residue diet for 3 days before the examination, followed by a liquid diet from midday on the day before the examination. The instructions given to the patient include a list of low-residue foods and suitable liquid foods. Clear fluids only are permitted on the morning of the examination.

Increased Fluid Intake

A large volume of liquid, 250 ml per hour for 8–10 hours, is suggested on the day preceding the examination.

Laxatives

Two laxatives are routinely given on the day before the examination; castor oil (35 ml) at noon and 16 mg magnesium sulphate at 4.00 p.m. The castor oil is much easier to take if it is mixed with concentrated orange juice.

Cleansing Enema

The cleansing enema should be performed in the x-ray department. No special equipment is required and 2,000 ml tap water, at or near body temperature, is administered (Miller 1975). The enema should be administered slowly at first, with the enema bag near the level of the couch. The bag is then gradually raised to increase the speed of administration, but it should never be raised more than 3 ft. above the couch. It the patient experiences spasm the tubing should not be clamped; rather than this the bag should be lowered to the level of the couch or lower to reduce the pressure. As the enema is administered the patient lies first in the prone position, then on the left side, then prone or supine, and finally on the right side. In this way gravity helps the column of water pass through the colon as far as the caecum. It is best to leave an interval of $1^1/_2$–2 h between the cleansing enema and the examination. This allows time for the patient to get rid of all residual fluid while the colon absorbs any fluid that the patient fails to evacuate.

Barium Suspension

The barium suspension used for the double-contrast barium enema examination should be capable of producing good homogeneous coating of the mucosa of the colon for sufficient time to allow radiographs to be obtained. This important aspect of the double-contrast barium enema examination has been neglected. The most suitable barium suspensions are those prepared by the manufacturers specifically for the double-contrast examination of the colon and delivered ready for use. While a number of these 'ready-to-use' barium suspensions are prepared by manufacturers in other countries there is as yet no such preparation available in the United Kingdom. Some of the barium preparations are supplied in the form of barium sulphate powder, and water has to be added to make a suspension. Others come in the form of a suspension that needs to be diluted by adding water.

Suspensions prepared in the department (by mixing barium sulphate powder with water) are unlikely to give consistently good results. There may be difficulty in getting the barium sulphate to suspend properly, as the local water supply has an effect on the performance of the suspension (Miller and Skucas 1977). If the water used is unsatisfactory, artefacts caused by flocculation, foaming, or bubble formation may cause problems. Variants in the local water supply are very important as the same barium sulphate could perform satisfactorily in one radiology department and not in another. Similarly, barium suspensions that require dilution with water before use can give inconsistent results.

Hypotonic Agent

Smooth muscle relaxants are necessary for good results because the colon can then be examined in a relaxed state, ensuring that small lesions can be seen. Hyoscine butylbromide (Buscopan) and glucagon are widely used for this purpose.

Hyoscine butylbromide is a quarternary ammonium synthesized from scopolamine (Ayre-Smith 1976). It is a ganglion-blocking agent, having no central action (unlike scopolamine). It causes only minor atropine-like side-effects unless doses of over 40 mg are employed. Higher doses lead to a significant incidence of side-effects such as dryness of the mucous membranes, mydriasis, palpitations, nausea, and headaches. Hyoscine butylbromide has its main action on the parasympathetically innervated visceral organs which contain smooth muscle. Hence its marked effect on the gastrointestinal tract. Hyoscine butylbromide is the drug of choice for the double-contrast barium enema examination of the colon; a dose of 20 mg IV is normally adequate. Contraindications to its use include heart failure, angina pectoris, prostatism, and glaucoma. The dose prescribed above would be unlikely to aggravate heart failure or angina or produce retention.

Glucagon, a straight-chain polypeptide derived from the alpha cells of the pancreatic islets of Langerhans, also inhibits gastrointestinal motility. It is now used in many centres as an agent for producing hypotonia during examinations of the colon (Miller et al. 1974). Nausea and vomiting can occur, but are rare with the small dose used for producing gastrointestinal hypotonia. Glucagon can provoke severe hypertension in patients with a phaeochromocytoma, and sensitization reactions can occur, although they are rare. The normal dose of glucagon used is 0.25–0.5 mg IV.

Examination Techniques

The double-contrast enema technique that is now used is based on the Malmö method (Welin 1958). The barium is introduced into the rectum with the patient lying horizontal on the fluoroscopy table. The flow of barium is started with the patient on the left side and the head of the barium column is observed intermittently at fluoroscopy. If the patient develops pain or discomfort during the introduction of the barium the bag containing the barium is lowered to reduce the intracolonic pressure. As the head of the barium column reaches the splenic flexure the patient lies prone or supine. When the barium reaches the proximal transverse colon the flow is stopped and the patient is sent to the toilet with instructions to evacuate as much barium as possible and to return to the x-ray room immediately. The alternative, used by many radiologists, is to drain the barium from the rectum and colon while the patient remains on the fluoroscopy table. More barium is evacuated if the patient goes to the toilet, and as a result the barium is more completely drained from the rectum and distal sigmoid colon.

Before air is insufflated, 20 mg hyoscine butylbromide (Buscopan) is injected IV. The air is then introduced into the rectum by means of a Higgenson's syringe. Air insufflation can be very uncomfortable if large amounts are introduced rapidly into the rectum. It is much better to obtain a continuous flow of air by insufflating small amounts quickly. Initially air is introduced with the patient lying prone. The ileocaecal valve is situated posteriorly, and when the patient is prone it is air, and not barium, that will pass into the terminal ileum when the caecum becomes distended. This prevents the sigmoid loops from being obscured by barium in the terminal ileum. If barium has not passed to the ascending colon, air insufflation is carried out initially with the patient on the right side.

When the colon is filled with air radiographs are obtained. A full-length prone view, a prone view of the sigmoid colon with the tube angled caudad 30° (Dysart and Stewart 1966), a full-length supine, a right decubitus, and a left decubitus view are taken with the overcouch tube. With the aid of fluoroscopy a lateral view of the rectum and a right anterior oblique view of the sigmoid colon are taken. The patient is then brought to an upright position and oblique views to open up the splenic flexure and the hepatic flexure are taken. This is followed by a full-size film with the patient upright. Other views and spot films are taken as required.

Radiological Appearances of Carcinoma of the Colon

Radiologically there are two principal appearances of primary carcinoma of the colon. Infiltrating lesions are the type most commonly seen. In some cases they are seen infiltrating and distorting part of the wall of the colon or rectum with destruction of the normal mucosal pattern (Fig. 1). At a more advanced stage the infiltrating carcinoma is seen as an annular growth involving the complete circumference of the colon and causing stenosis (Fig. 2). The normal mucosal pattern of the narrowed segment is completely destroyed, the lumen is irregular, and there is often shouldering of the upper and lower margins of the tumour. The other radiological manifestation of carcinoma of the colon is as a polypoid lesion. Polypoid lesions are fairly large and irregular (Fig. 3), and can fill most of the lumen of the segment of colon involved. It may be impossible to differentiate benign polyps (Fig. 4) from carcinoma on the basis of the radiological appearances alone. Malignant change is present in 46% of colonic polyps greater than 2 cm in size, in 9.5% of those between 1 and 2 cm, and in 1.3% of those less than 1 cm in size (Morson 1974).

Radiological features of polypoid lesions that suggest malignancy include dimpling or indentation at the base, an irregular surface, and an increase in size (Welin and Welin 1976). When the breadth of the base of the polyp is greater than the height and the outline of the polyp *en face* is oval the growth is more likely to be malignant.

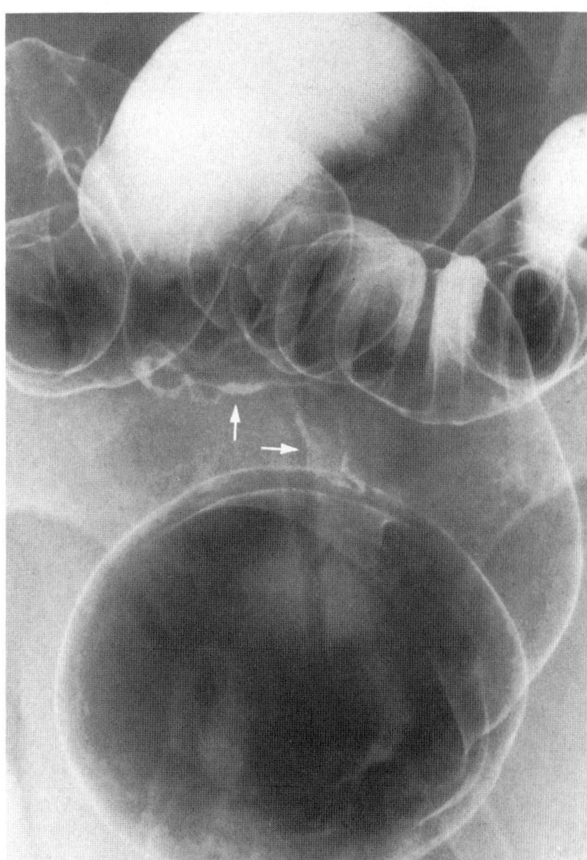

Fig. 1. Infiltrating carcinoma. This 50-year-old man complained of motions with blood on the surface. Three polyps, removed at sigmoidoscopy 5 years previously, proved to be villous adenomas. Sigmoidoscopy was performed first and no lesion was seen. This prone angled view shows slight infiltration and irregularity of part of the wall of the distal sigmoid colon (*arrows*) and it was the only radiographic view that showed the abnormal area. At operation a carcinoma, that proved to be a well-differentiated adenocarcinoma (Dukes' B) was found. Reproduced by courtesy of HM+M Publishers

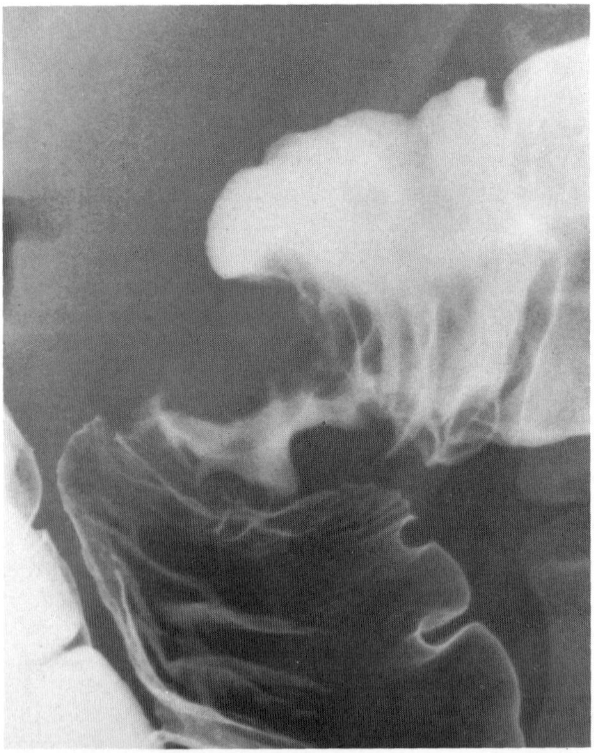

Fig. 2. Infiltrating carcinoma. An annular carcinoma is seen in the transverse colon. There is shouldering of the margins, an irregular, narrowed lumen, and destruction of the normal mucosal pattern

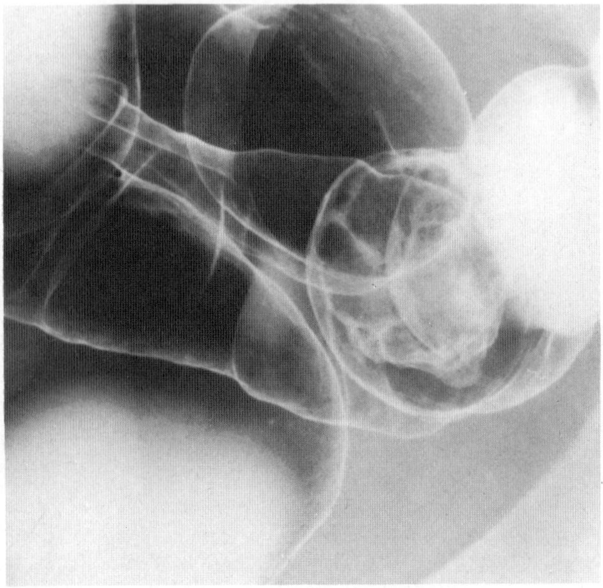

Fig. 3. Polypoid carcinoma. The patient, a 66-year-old woman, had a barium enema performed after presenting with left iliac fossa pain. A well-differentiated adenocarcinoma was found at operation, infiltrating the inner margin of the main muscle coat but no deeper

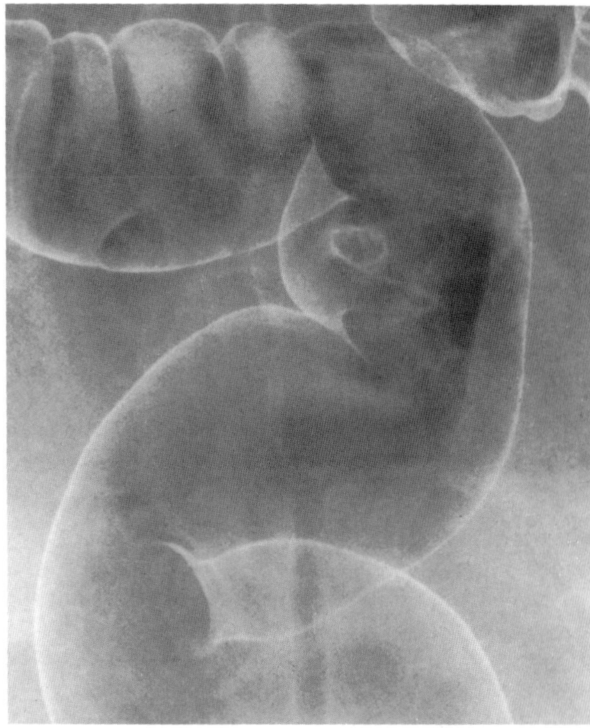

Fig. 4. Polyp in sigmoid colon. The patient, a 65-year-old man, presented with rectal bleeding. A small, sessile polyp with a slightly irregular margin is seen in the distal sigmoid colon. This was removed at sigmoidoscopy and on histological examination proved to be a tubular adenoma

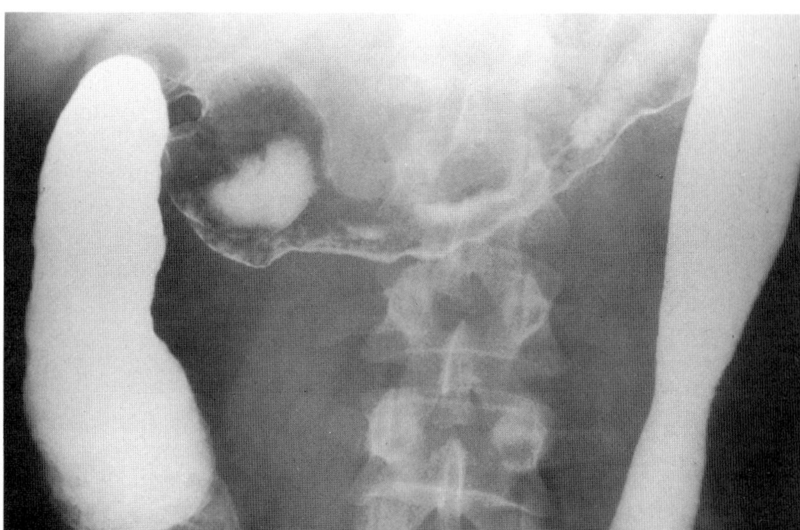

Fig. 5. Carcinoma complicating ulcerative colitis. This 40-year-old man presented with bloody diarrhoea and weight loss. He had a 7-year history of ulcerative colitis. An extensive infiltrating carcinoma of the transverse colon is seen. At operation a carcinoma extending from the hepatic flexure to the splenic flexure was confirmed It was adherent to the pancreas; many seedlings were present in the peritoneum and it was inoperable. Histology of the peritoneal seedlings showed a poorly differentiated mucus-secreting adenocarcinoma. Reproduced by courtesy of HM+M Publishers

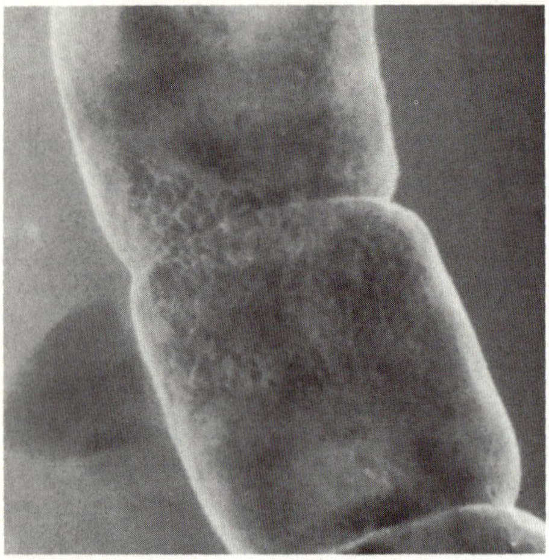

Fig. 6. Epithelial dysplasia in ulcerative colitis. An irregular nodular area is seen in a segment of the descending colon. The patient, a 24-year-old woman, was known to have had ulcerative colitis for 8 years. Colonoscopy was carried out and epithelial dysplasia was confirmed on histological examination of the biopsies obtained. Reproduced by courtesy of HM+M Publishers

Five percent of patients with carcinoma of the colon or rectum will have more than one cancer (Morson and Dawson 1979). It is, therefore, very important to look for evidence of more than one cancer when performing barium studies of the colon. Patients who have a cancer of the rectum or sigmoid colon detected on digital examination or sigmoidoscopy should have a full double-contrast enema to evaluate the remainder of the colon. It is not uncommon to find adenomatous polyps present in the colon of patients with cancer. Multiple tumours, ademomas, or adenocarcinomas were present synchronously in 20% of the patients in one survey (Muto et al. 1975).

There is a high incidence of cancer of the colon in familial polyposis coli, a condition which is inherited as a dominant Mendelian character. The double-contrast barium enema is important for examining close relatives of patients who have this condition.

An increased incidence of carcinoma of the colon occurs in patients with ulcerative colitis. Extensive colonic involvement, duration of the disease for more than 10 years, and an early age of onset increase the risk of developing cancer. There are features which may distinguish cancer in colitis from ordinary colonic cancer (Morson and Dawson 1979). In ulcerative colitis the cancers are often multiple and arise predominantly on the left side of the colon. They are often flat and infiltrating with an ill-defined edge (Fig. 5). There is also a higher incidence of high grade and colloid carcinomas.

The detection of severe dysplasia can identify patients with a high risk of developing cancer. Characteristic radiological abnormalities have been identified in areas of mucosa associated with histologically proven dysplasia (Frank et al. 1978). These appearances include nodularity and irregular areas with sharply angled edges which may represent enlarged *areae colonicae* (Fig. 6). Demonstration of these changes is an indication for endoscopic examination and biopsy of the suggestive area.

Barium Enema and Colonoscopy

The introduction and widespread use of colonoscopy has led to the more accurate diagnosis of colonic cancer and polyps. The main advantages of colonoscopy are that polyps can be removed and biopsies can be obtained from polypoid lesions and from the mucosa of the colon. Digital examination, sigmoidoscopy, and barium enema remain the initial diagnostic procedures in patients with suspected colonic disease. There are limiting factors to the accuracy of colonoscopy. Even with a clean colon lesions may be missed at the flexures because of the sharp angulation. In about 10% of patients the colonoscopist will fail to reach the caecum. Miller and Lehman (1978) collected 54 patients with radiographically detected polypoid colonic lesions that were missed by sigmoidoscopy or colonoscopy. In each patient the endoscopist had reached or passed beyond the area of the lesions, but failed to identify the polypoid tumour. A patient was noticed recently who had a small carcinoma of the caecum that had been detected on the initial radiographic examination and subsequently proved at operation, and had been missed at two colonoscopy examinations. Both colonoscopy examinations were performed after the barium study, with full knowledge of the radiographic findings, and on each occasion the endoscopist assumed he had reached and adequately visualized the caecum.

When a high-quality radiological study suggests a polypoid lesion that is not confirmed at endoscopy, it should not be assumed that the lesion is an artefact (Laufer et al. 1976). Endoscopy and double-contrast barium radiology are complementary and their combined diagnostic accuracy exceeds that of either technique (Miller and Lehman 1978).

References

Ayre-Smith G (1976) Hyoscine-*N*-butylbromide (Buscopan) as a duodenal relaxant in tubeless duodenography. Acta Radiol [Diagn] (Stockh) 17: 701–713

Dysart DN, Stewart HR (1966) Special angled roentgenography of lesions of the recto-sigmoid: five-year survey. AJR 96: 285–291

Frank PH, Riddell RH, Feczko PJ, Levin B (1978) Radiological detection of colonic dysplasia (precarcinoma) in chronic ulcerative colitis. Gastrointest Radiol 3: 209–219

Kellett MJ, Zboralske FF, Margulis AR (1977) Per oral pneumocolon examination of the ileo-caecal region. Gastrointest Radiol 1: 361–365

Laufer I, Smith NCW, Mullens JE (1976) The radiological demonstration of colorectal polyps undetected by endoscopy. Gastroenterology 70: 167–170

Miller RE (1975) The cleansing enema. Radiology 117: 483–485

Miller RE (1976) The clean colon. Gastroenterology 70: 289–290

Miller RE, Lehman G (1978) Polypoid colonic lesions undetected by endoscopy. Radiology 129: 295–297

Miller RE, Skucas J (1977) Radiographic contrast agents. University Park Press, Baltimore

Miller RE, Chernish SM, Skucas J, Rosenak BD, Rodda BE (1974) Hypotonic colon examination with glucagon. Radiology 113: 555–562

Morson BC (1974) The polyp cancer sequence in the large bowel. J R Soc Med 67: 451–457

Morson BC, Dawson IMP (1979) Gastrointestinal pathology. Blackwell Scientific, Oxford

Muto T, Bussey HJR, Morson BC (1975) The evolution of cancer of the colon and rectum. Cancer 36: 2251–2270

Saunders CG, MacEwen DW (1971) Delay in diagnosis of colonic cancer – a continuing challenge. Radiology 101: 207–208

Welin S (1958) Modern trends in diagnostic roentgenology of the colon. Br J Radiol 31: 453–464

Welin S, Welin G (1976) The double-contrast examination of the colon. Experiences with the Welin modification. Thieme, Stuttgart

Early Diagnosis and Detection

J. D. Hardcastle and K. D. Vellacott

Department of Surgery, Queens Medical Centre, University of Nottingham, Nottingham NG7 2UH, United Kingdom

Survival from colorectal cancer is dependent upon the stage of disease at the time of diagnosis or treatment. In a recent study from a regional hospital, Oxford, the corrected 5-year survival following detection in Dukes' stage A was 100%, in stage B 58%, in stage C 27.1%, and in stage D 5.5% (Gill and Morris 1978). Patients admitted with this condition and emergency treatment for obstruction or perforation have a hospital mortality of 24%, compared with only 3.6% for patients treated electively (Till 1977). The mortality is particularly high in the elderly requiring emergency colonic resections (Boyd et al. 1980).

It is clear from all series that patients with stage A colorectal cancers have an excellent prognosis and it is therefore disappointing that these only constitute 5.7%–14.3% of the total operated cases in England and Wales (Lockhart-Mummery et al. 1976; Gill and Morris 1978).

Improvements in surgical and anaesthetic techniques have made little impression on the 5-year survival results (Clarke et al. 1980) and it seems logical therefore that efforts should be made to detect tumours at an early stage.

Does the detection of asymptomatic tumours result in an increase in the number of Dukes' stage A tumours found, and what evidence is there that the overall survival is improved?

The results of a long-term clinical study at the Cancer Detection Center at the University of Minnesota suggests that this is likely (Gilbertsen and Nelms 1978). Over a 28-year period, 21,150 men and women were examined by annual proctosigmoidoscopy. Twenty-seven adenocarcinomas were found on the first examination. At each yearly examination all adenomatous polyps were removed, and only 13 further cancers were detected. The incidence of developing cancers was only 15% of that anticipated from epidemiological data, and 80% of these cancers were confined to the submucosa. The 5-year survival of the 13 patients found to have adenocarcinomas was 85%, including one postoperative death and one patient who died of pancreatic cancer. In 22% of these patients the tumour was shown to have spread distally, as against 55% in a group of symptomatic patients. Of the 27 adenocarcinomas detected at the first examination, 25 had been followed-up for 5 years and there were 16 survivors (64%), twice the overall 5-year survival reported for symptomatic cancer (Gill and Morris 1978).

In a collaborative study involving the Memorial Sloan-Kettering Cancer Center and the Strang Clinic, New York, 21,961 persons were studied by proctosigmoidoscopy and faecal occult blood testing. Most of these subjects were asymptomatic but 7% had minor symptoms. Thirty-two cancers were detected on first examination, and 27 on subsequent examinations. In all, 59% of the cancers detected at the initial examination

Recent Results in Cancer Research, Vol. 83

and 7% of these found at the subsequent examination were staged as Dukes' A or B (Winawer et al. 1980).

Evolution of Colorectal Cancer from Polyps

There is clinical, pathological, and epidemiological evidence to suggest that the majority of colorectal cancers arise in benign adenomatous polpys.

The geographical distribution of colonic adenomas around the world closely parallels the distribution of colorectal cancer, with a high prevalence in western countries (Correa et al. 1977). The introduction of the fiberoptic colonoscope has provided further support for this, in that the distribution of colonic adenomas found at colonoscopy is the same as for cancer (Gillespie et al. 1979; Wolff and Shinya 1978). Autopsies on 14,000 African Bantu, in whome there is a very low incidence of colorectal cancer, revealed no adenomatous polyps (Bremner and Ackerman 1970). Hyperplastic (or metaplastic) polyps have no malignant potential (Fenoglio and Lane 1974) but adenomatous polyps, which may be tubular, tubulo-villous or villous, are premalignant (Wolff and Shinya 1978). The risk of malignant change is related to the size of the adenoma and its histology. Only about 1% of adenomas under 1 cm in size undergo malignant change (Morson 1974; Welch 1979). This proportion rises to about 10% in those between 1 and 2 cm in diameter and is nearly 50% in those over 2 cm in size. This suggests that as adenomas grow the cancer risk rises. The histological features are important, the villous pattern involving a higher chance of malignancy. In situ carcinoma and invasive carcinoma has been demonstrated in 7% and 0.6%, respectively, of tubular adenomas as against 19% and 4% in tubulovillous adenomas (Enterline 1974).

Those patients who have a cancer resected and are found to have adenomatous polyps present in the resected specimen have an increased risk of developing a second primary tumour (Morson 1976). In the surveillance of patients over 8 years 2.7% of those with known adenomatous polyps developed cancer, as opposed to none in a group with no polyps (Brahme et al. 1974).

In a series of malignant tumours, 14.2% showed evidence of contiguous benign tumour and in those with invasion of the submucosa only, 60% were associated with adenomatous tissue, suggesting the increasing growth destroys the benign tissue (Morson 1966).

How long an adenomatous polyp takes to become malignant is difficult to ascertain, but it may be as long as 10–15 years. A single polyp observed at the Mayo Clinic developed malignant change after 15 years (Mayo and de Castro 1956). Three out of four solitary adenomatous polyps studied at St. Mark's Hospital developed cancer within 12.5 years (Morson 1976).

Familial polyposis coli demonstrates the development of cancer from pre-existing adenomas. The average age at diagnosis of polyposis coli without malignant change is 27 years, while it is 39 years in those family members who present with cancer (Bussey 1975). The condition is inherited as an autosomal dominant trait with an almost 100% risk of eventually developing carcinoma. (Alm and Licznerski 1973).

The peak incidence for colorectal cancer is in the 60–70 age group (Falterman et al. 1974). The frequency of hyperplastic polyps in autopsy specimens is 20% of all cases with no age variance. Adenomas, on the other hand, increase in frequency with age (Eide and Stalsberg 1978).

It seems logical therefore that to reduce the incidence of colorectal cancer and to improve the mortality, adenomatous polyps need to be detected before they develop invasive cancers as well as cancers at an early stage of development.

Screening for Colorectal Tumours

The ideal screening test would be one that is sufficiently sensitive to detect the majority of tumours without a high false-positive rate. The only two practical methods at present available are proctosigmoidoscopy and faecal occult blood testing.

Proctosigmoidoscopy

Approximately 42% of all colorectal cancers occur within range of the rigid 25 cm sigmoidoscope (Falterman et al. 1974). Conventional rigid sigmoidoscopy is easy to perform and has proved useful in detecting adenomatous polyps (Payne 1976).

Studies in the United States with rigid sigmoidoscopy examination have been conducted in motivated persons attending screening clinics. In persons over 40 years of age the rate of detection of invasive cancers was 0.12% (Moertel et al. 1966), 0.13% at the Minnesota Cancer Detection Center (Gilbertsen 1974), and 0.12% at the Strang Institute (Sherlock and Winawer 1977). However, the detection of polyps is much higher, varying from 3% to 4% of persons screened over 40 years of age (Moertel et al. 1966; Payne 1976).

In conventional rigid sigmoidoscopy the distance passed with an adequate view is dependent on whether a preparatory enema is given. In our own studies on 60 patients we found the distance passed without any preparation was 16.8 ± 5.0 cm (Mean $\pm$ SD) with an adequate view in 77% of patients. When a phosphate enema was given the sigmoidoscope was passed 20.0 ± 4.4 cm, with a good view in 100% of patients. The majority of carcinomas and adenomatous polyps occur on the left side of the colon. In a study of 1,049 colonic adenomas, 97% of which were removed endoscopically, it was found that two-thirds of the larger adenomas 2 cm or more in diameter were situated in the sigmoid colon. Of those containing invasive carcinoma (4.8% of the total polyps), 94% were in the sigmoid or lower part of the descending colon (Gillespie et al. 1979). This distribution emphasizes the potential value of the 60 cm fiberoptic sigmoidoscope, as most of these lesions would be revealed by this examination. It has advantages over the conventional long colonoscope, in that it can be done quickly without sedation and a phosphate enema is the only preparation needed.

Comparison of flexible and rigid sigmoidsocopy has shown a 3.2 times greater yield of information with the flexible instrument (Marks et al. 1979). The fiberoptic sigmoidoscope can be inserted the full 60 cm in 55%–62% of cases (Bohlman et al. 1977; Marks et al. 1979). When 200 asymptomatic patients over the age of 40 were examined, 53 polyps were found in 39 patients, 22 of the polyps being greater than 0.5 cm in diameter. More than half were beyond the reach of the rigid sigmoidoscope (Lipshutz et al. 1979).

Preparation with a single enema is adequate in over 90% of cases, and the time taken to perform the examination is only a few minutes longer than for rigid sigmoidoscopy (Bohlman et al. 1977; Manier 1978; Foster et al. 1981).

Because of the ease with which the investigation is carried out and minimal discomfort to most patients, flexible sigmoidoscopy should probably be the first investigation of choice in investigating patients found to be faecal occult blood-positive in screening studies (Hardcastle et al. 1980).

Faecal Occult Blood Testing

The theoretically ideal faecal occult blood test should be simple and easy to perform. It should be sufficiently sensitive to detect small amounts of blood, but not so sensitive as to detect normal daily blood loss. It should not be influenced by an ordinary diet or commonly used medicines, and should be applicable to stored faeces (Needham and Simpson 1952). None of the available chemical tests fulfils these requirements.

Gastrointestinal blood loss may become apparent with as little as 50 ml resulting in tarry stools (Irons and Kirsner 1965). Normal blood loss has been estimated in healthy individuals by means of radioactive chromium red cell labelling methods and was found to be in the range of 1–2 ml per day (Roche et al. 1957; Ebaugh et al. 1958; Jones 1958; Cameron 1960). These studies indicated that the upper limit of normal is 2.0 mg haemoglobin per gram of stool, assuming a 150 g stool per day in a patient with a haemoglobin of 15 gm/100 ml (Morris et al. 1976).

A different method, a quantitative benzidine test, has yielded similar results have been obtained (Ebaugh and Beeken 1959). The daily blood loss may be increased by ingestion of such drugs as salicylates (Grossman et al. 1961).

Most of the chemical tests are dependent on the oxidation of a phenolic compound to a quinone structure which yields a blue dye by an intermolecular reaction (Harvey 1956). It is the haematin component of haemoglobin that catalyses the oxidation of chromagenic indicators such as benzidine, orthotolidine, and guaiac, resulting in a blue or green colour (Thornton and Illingworth 1955). The oxidation is facilitated by hydrogen peroxide; naturally occurring peroxidases, which have a similar structure to haematin, may also act as catalysts. The sensitive chemical tests may therefore have false-positive reactions due to haemoglobin present in animal meats and blood puddings, and also to vegetable peroxidases. Conversely, ascorbic acid may be a cause of false-negative results because of its reducing action interfering with the quinone reaction (Jaffe et al. 1975).

Varying results have been obtained in clinical studies with benzidine, orthotolidine and guaiac tests. Generally the benzidine and orthotolidine tests are far too sensitive and the original guaiac tests were too inaccurate (Irons and Kirsner 1956).

In recent years several chemical tests based on benzidine and orthotolidine have been withdrawn since the Chester Beatty Institute and Harlow Industrial Health Service (1966) suggested a carcinogenic hazard in handling aromatic amines.

To improve the accuracy of the guaiac test, a specially prepared guaiac-impregnated electrophoresis filter paper, Haemoccult (Eaton Laboratories, England), was developed and made into a slide suitable for patients to use at home. To reduce the incidence of false-positives, a meat-free high-residue diet was suggested before the test was done. To increase the true-positive rate it was advised that three consecutive stools should be tested (Greegor 1971).

In a study comparing the sensitivity of guaiac reagent, orthotolidine (Hematest), and the modified guaiac reagent (Haemoccult), in which haemoglobin in stool was estimated by ^{51}Cr red cells assay, false-positives occurred in 72%, 76%, and 12% of tests, respectively (Morris et al. 1976). This showed Haemoccult to be the least sensitive test but subject to less false-positive reactions, where false-positives occur with a blood loss of less than 2 mg haemoglobin per gram of stool. All these methods are subject to an observer error in recording a colour change (Ostrow et al. 1973).

Storage of stools for as little as 3 days led to an increased guaiac reactivity, often with conversion of a negative reaction to a positive. The reverse occurred with Hematest. By contrast, Haemoccult is little affected by storage in the test envelope at room temperature (Ostrow et al. 1973), though a diminished frequency of positive reactions with Haemoccult has also been reported (Morris et al. 1976).

Recently a more sensitive guaiac test, Fecatest (Finn pipette, Finland), has been introduced. This is sensitive enough to detect as little as 2–3 mg haemoglobin per gram of homogenized stool (Aldercreutz et al. 1980). However, when tested on 150 unselected patients Fecatest was found to be positive in 50% immediately and in 70% after storage. It was concluded that Fecatest could not be recommended for screening for colonic tumours (Beretta et al. 1978).

Other chemical methods have also been developed recently. Jaffe and Zierdt (1979) developed a faecal extraction test with a lower false-positive rate than Haemoccult. Peroheme-40, another chemical method dependent on the peroxidase activity of haemoglobin, has the disadvantage of requiring dietary restriction to avoid false-positives (Krasner et al. 1975).

When gastrointestinal blood loss does not exceed 2 ml per day, approximately 10% of stool specimens collected from patients not on dietary restricition will be Haemoccult-positive (Stroehlein et al. 1976), this being reduced to about 2% by dietary restriction (Basset and Goulston 1980). For meat to cause a false-positive result large amounts need to be digested, 480 g causing a positive Fecatest while 240 g meat per day gives negative results (Brault and Favre 1979).

The Haemoccult test is the method most widely used a present. However, it is not known exactly to what degree cancers bleed. From early studies it seems that the majority of adenomatous polyps do not bleed, as most are negative on all occult blood tests (Cameron 1960). Blood is not distributed evenly throughout faeces, and it is therefore important that more than one test is performed and two different areas of each stool are tested. In addition, if faeces is added to water the Haemoccult sensitivity is increased when the suspension is tested (Rosenfield et al. 1979).

A blood loss of more than 10 ml is required to obtain over 90% positive Haemoccult tests as estimated by ^{51}Cr-labelled blood (Strohlein et al. 1976).

The amount of bleeding from the upper gastrointestinal tract required to give a positive Haemoccult is much larger than from the colon. Subjects given labelled blood orally had only one positive reaction when 30 ml was ingested, despite the presence of a concentration of 23 mg haemoglobin in the stool (Ranson et al. 1980). These findings have been confirmed by other workers, who have shown that 30 ml ingested blood is necessary for a positive Haemoccult test, though Fecatest gave some positive results with as little as 5–10 ml of ingested blood (Parkins and Barrison 1981).

It is difficult to compare the sensitivities of various tests as there is poor correlation between in vitro results involving the addition of blood or haemolysates to faeces and in vivo results (Aldercreutz et al. 1980).

These are several sources of error in the chemical tests. These are due to in, adequate samples, absence of preparatory diet, sample stored too long, use of certain medications, samples taken from the same area of stool, and the test being performed on only one occasion.

False Negatives with Haemoccult Testing

Very few studies have been done to ascertain the false-negative rate for proven tumours with Haemoccult slide testing. However, the rate can be calculated from some studies. Table 1 shows the false-negative results in studies of polyps and cancers. Two studies (Katon et al. 1977; Lipshutz et al. 1979) investigated the results of Haemoccult testing on patients who were subsequently found to have benign polyps on fiberoptic sigmoidoscopy. Many of these polyps were small and in Lipshutz's study 15.6% were hyperplastic, which accounts for the very high false-negative rate. The studies of Winawer et al. (1980), Ribet et al. (1980), Rozen et al. (1980), and Gnauk (1980) were screening studies which also incorporated sigmoidoscopy examinations. The polyps in Gnauk's study were all greater than 0.5 cm in diameter and all were adenomatous. The 84 of 214 polyps that were negative were only those that were found within reach of a sigmoidoscope. The result reported does not take into account the lesions higher in the bowel which were asymptomatic. It seems likely, therefore, that the false-negative rate for adenomatous polyps is at the very least 39% but is more likely to be in the order of 60%–70%.

Radiochromium methods used in 44 patients with polyps greater than 1.5 cm in diameter suggest that the average daily blood loss for polyps in the rectosigmoid and descending colon was 1.36 ± 0.14 ml, as against 1.28 ± 0.31 ml per day for those in the right side of the colon. A total of 1,474 Haemoccult tests were performed, and only 583 (39.5%) were positive (Herzog et al. 1981).

As far as cancer patients are concerned only a small number with proven cancer have been tested. The patients whose results were false-negative in the screening surveys, as with the polyps, were those that were subsequently diagnosed as having cancer. Those who were negative on Haemoccult testing and had no symptoms were not investigated further apart from sigmoidoscopy.

Songster et al. (1980) tested 150 patients, but not all were tested on each of 3 days, some having only one test done. In this group 60% were negative. Doran et al. (to be published) tested 50 patients, who were in hospital with proven cancers, over 6 consecutive days. On the first 3 days of testing 30% were negative.

Table 1. False-negatives with Heamoccult testing

Reference	Type of study	Number of cancers negative	Number of polyps negative
Winawer et al. 1977a	Screening	2/9 (22%)	15/38 (39.5%)
Katon et al. 1977	Fiberoptic sigmoidoscopy		15/19 (80%)
Lipshutz et al. 1979	Fiberoptic sigmoidoscopy		30/36 (83.3%)
Ostrow et al. 1973	Proven tumours	3/7 (42.8%)	3/6 (50%)
Colin et al. 1978	Proven tumours	4/17 (23.5%)	4/23 (17.4%)
Winawer et al. 1980	Screening	25%	16/21 (76%)
Ribet et al. 1980	Screening	2/3 (66.6%)	23/27 (85%)
Rozen et al. 1980	Screening		8/13 (61.5%)
Gnauk 1980	Screening	12/93 (13%)	84/214 (39%)
Songster et al. 1980	Proven tumours	90/150 (60%)	
Doran et al. to be puplished	Proven tumours	15/50 (30%)	

The success of a screening test is dependent on the compliance of those to whom it is offered. Persons who volunteer for screening have a high compliance rate, 80%–91.5% (Glober and Peskoe 1974; Winawer et al. 1980), as do those from institutions or military establishments (Miller and Knight 1977). A high compliance may also be obtained by publicity in the form of meetings, newspapers, radio, and television advertising (Richardson 1977; Bralow 1979). However, even with publicity some studies have an acceptance rate as low as 26% (Winchester et al. 1980).

In the United States, when test kits were distributed without warning through the post to the adult population, the compliance was only 15% (James 1977). In a pilot study in the United Kingdom, 1638 invitations were sent out to persons over the age of 45 registered in one general practice. The overall compliance was found to be 45%, being 65% in the 45–60 age group, but as low as 25% in those over 75 years. The results of this study were that 29 (3.8%) were positive, and two carcinomas were found along with three adenomatous polyps. Eighteen were subsequently negative on repeat occult blood testing (Hardcastle et al. 1980).

Table 2 summarizes the results obtained from screening studies around the world with Haemoccult testing. Those studies with high compliance rates were conducted in persons attending screening clinics. Only three of the studies, those of Hardcastle et al. (1980), Million et al. (1980), and Farrands et al. (to be published), were performed in England: in Nottingham, Salford, and Frome.

These studies and others (Gilbertsen et al. 1980; Winawer et al. 1980) show that faecal occult blood testing on those over 40 years will detect 1.3–4.5 cancers per 1,000 of the population screened. In addition, in the study from Minnesota (Gilbertsen et al. 1980) 49 of 75 gastrointestinal cancers (65%) were Dukes' stage A tumours.

In New York 59% of 71 colon cancers detected were Dukes' stage A or B, as against only 33% in a control group (Winawer et al. 1980). There is therefore increasing evidence that the use of faecal occult blood testing to detect asymptomatic cancers may result in the treatment of a high proportion of early stage cancers.

Immunological Methods

The basic principle of detecting haemoglobin in stool samples is based on the fact that haemoglobin is present in extremely high concentrations in blood. Immunological methods specifically designed to identify human haemoglobin should therefore remove most of the causes of the false-positive reactions obtained with chemical tests. By developing monospecific antisera to human haemoglobin, faecal samples can be tested with radial immunodiffusion plates (Barrows et al. 1978; Songster et al. 1980). The sensitivity of immunological tests for haemoglobin appears to be better than that of the guaiac peroxidase tests. While loss of antigenic activity of haemoglobin in faeces was found to be significant, a similar loss of reactivity is present with guaiac tests. No cross reaction with animal haemoglobins was found except with the rabbit (Barrows et al. 1978).

These methods were used to test a least one stool sample from each of 150 consecutive patients. Both Haemoccult and the immunochemical tests gave negative results in 29% of cases; 50% of rectal lesions and 25% of right-sided colonic lesions were negative. Occult bleeding was found in 40% by Haemoccult and 63% by the immunochemical test. This study suggested that immunochemical methods to detect colorectal bleeding from carcinoma are more sensitive than existing chemical methods (Songster et al.

Table 2. Screening studies with Haemoccult slide test

Reference	Number offered test	Number accepted	% Acceptance	% Positive	Number of cancers detected	Number of polyps
1. Glober and Peskoe 1974	1,682	1,539	91.5	23.7	3	3
2. Hastings 1974	2,272	1,835	80.0	6.2	5	–
3. Durst et al. 1976	4,000	1,125	28.0	5.8	4	4
4. Ross and Johnson 1976	1,187	1,103	93.0	7.0	4	–
5. Miller and Knight 1977	2,332	2,205	94.5	2.8	3	7
6. Richardson 1977	1,038	885	85.0	6.1	0	4
7. Jorge et al. 1977	1,437	1,150	80.0	4.6	7	4
8. Frühmorgen and Demling 1978	6,007	5,015	83.5	2.7	13	83
9. Withers and James 1978	1,050	–	–	10.6	4	25
10. Helfrick and Petrucci 1979	49,157	19,707	40.0	4.6	15	18
11. Norfleet and Roberts 1979	492	236	50.0	6.4	0	5
12. Spinelli et al. 1979	5,954	5,015	–	1.75	10	9
13. Samec 1979	5,323	3,887	73.0	4.12	12	23
14. Otto et al. 1979	8,727	–	–	3.2	27	35
15. Bralow 1979	3,798	–	79.0	10.9	7	11
16. Hardcastle et al. 1980	1,638	713	45.0	3.8	2	4
17. Winchester et al. 1980	54,101	14,074	26.0	4.4	27	40
18. Siba 1980	3,791	–	–	2.2	6	18
19. Schwartz et al. 1980	3,477,382	–	–	1.1	332	–
20. Winawer et al. 1980	13,127	9,709	74.0	2.5	43	–
21. Gilbertsen et al. 1980	48,000	–	–	1.8	72	271
22. Gnauk 1980	16,100	–	–	3.3	76	106
23. Million et al. 1980	3,481	1,179	33.9	2.7	2	3
24. Farrands et al. to be published	8,925	2,439	27.2	5.08	4	8

1980). As no dietary restriction is necessary they would simplify mass screening studies of asymptomatic populations. However, the methods in which radial immunodiffusion is used involve a 24–48 h delay before interpretation of the results, which would make it difficult to utilize on a large scale. An immunofluorescent test more suitable for population screening has recently been developed (Vellacott et al. 1981b). The test is dependent on fluorescein-labelled antihaemoglobin binding with haemoglobin in a faecal suspension. The unbound fluoresceinated antibody is subsequently bound to a membrane impregnated with haemoglobin, the fluorescence of which is recorded by means of a fluorometer.

Recently it has been shown that immunological tests do not react to upper gastrointestinal blood loss, possibly due to loss of antigenicity of haemoglobin because of digestive enzymes (Ostrow 1981). If this finding is confirmed the combination of chemical and immunological tests will be able to distinguish between upper and lower gastrointestinal blood loss with resultant saving in other investigations.

Tumour-Associated Products in Faeces

Colonoscope lavage of colonic adenomas, adenocarcinomas and normal controls has shown high levels of CEA to be present by Winawer et al. (1977b). This group studied 12 normal patients with no detectable colonic pathology, 9 with adenomatous polyps of less than 1 cm diameter, 26 with adenomatous polyps larger than 1 cm diameter, and 11 with histologically proven adenocarcinomas. Patients with polyps larger than 1 cm in diameter and those with adenocarcinomas had mean levels of CEA that were significantly higher than those of the normal controls, and those of patients with polyps less than 1 cm diameter. Using similar techniques, we have also shown high levels of CEA in the lavage fluid of patients with adenomatous polyps greater than 1 cm in diameter, inflammatory bowel disease, and colonic cancers compared with a group of patients with no gastrointestinal pathology. In addition, the colonic cancers appeared to be associated with higher levels than the rectal cancers.

In a separate study CEA was estimated in the colonic lavage of persons at risk of developing large-bowel cancer. Groups looked at consisted of hereditary polyposis families, both symptomatic and asymptomatic relatives, cancer-prone families, and 25 individuals with no increased risk. CEA was found to be significantly higher in the polyposis group than in the control individuals but was not raised in the individuals studied from cancer-prone families (Poleski et al. 1978).

CEA, however, is also produced by normal colonic mucosa. With a purely qualitative test the antigen was found to be present in the faeces of 5 of 10 healthy individuals and 10 of 11 cases of colonic cancer. Therefore any test must be quantitative to distinguish between normal and those with malignancy (Freed and Taylor 1972). Quantitative tests for CEA in the faeces of patients with colorectal cancer have shown higher levels than in healthy volunteers, though all the volunteers had CEA present in their faeces. The faecal CEA levels did not correlate with either the Dukes' staging or serum CEA levels (Fujimoto et al. 1979). In addition, in 14 patients treated by surgical resection, the faecal CEA levels clearly decreased after operation. In another study colonic mucus was obtained by suction through a sigmoidoscope distant from the site of a cancer. Of 23 patients with colonic carcinoma, all were found to have increased levels of CEA in the mucus. A high proportion of patients with gastric and pancreatic carcinomas were also found to have high levels in the fluids near the tumours (Molnar et al. 1976). Other CEA-like glycoproteins have also been identified in normal colon tissue and faeces (Rogers and Keep 1980; Kuroki et al. 1981), as have antigens in benign and malignant colonic tumours and in the mucosal cells adjacent to the tumours (Kawasaki and Kimito 1974; Bara et al. 1980). It has also been shown that abnormal sialomucins are secreted by colonic carcinomas and from the neighbouring but histologically normal mucosa, and the amount of mucosa producing abnormal mucins is directly related to the stage of the tumour (Filipe and Branfoot 1974; Greaves et al. 1980).

Tumour Markers in Blood

No specific tumour marker for colorectal cancer has been identified. Carcinoembryonic antigen (CEA) is raised in a variety of benign and malignant conditions and is of no value in the early detection of colorectal cancer. In 26 Dukes' stage A colorectal cancer patients we have studied, only one patient had elevated levels of CEA and none of 64 patients with benign adenomatous polyps had elevated levels.

The development of antibodies to purified CEA has enabled radiolabelled antibody to be used for localization of CEA-containing tumours. In nude mice bearing heterografts of human carcinomas, it was shown that immunoabsorbent purified goat anti-CEA antibodies were capable of specific localization in vivo into CEA-containing tumours, and that the radiolabelled antibodies could be detected by external scanning (Mach et al. 1974). Studies in man have confirmed localization in tumours (Goldenberg et al. 1980), but despite demonstrating specificity the antibody-derived radioactivity in the tumours is very small compared with the injected dose. The present scanning techniques show that this method of tumour detection is not yet clinically useful (Mach et al. 1980).

That tumour-associated antigens might exist, however, has been demonstrated by the study of circulating immune complexes, which have been shown to be increased in colorectal cancer, including early-stage disease, as well as in patients with adenomatous polyps (Vellacott et al. 1981a).

Conclusions

The overall prognosis of colorectal cancer has not improved over the past 20 years. Cancers detected at an early stage of disease, however, have an excellent 5-year survival rate. Persons with no symptoms who are found to have cancer have a higher chance of having the disease at an early stage (Dukes' A) than patients with symptoms. There is also increasing evidence that large adenomatous or villous polyps are premalignant lesions. Screening studies to detect these lesions in asymptomatic people should result in an improved prognosis, particularly at it is estimated that it may take from 10 to 20 years for a benign polyp to become a cancer.

Present methods of screening asymptomatic persons involve proctosigmoidoscopy and testing for blood in the stool. The ideal method would be a blood test to identify a tumour-related product, but at present none has been identified. There is evidence, however, that tumours may secrete antigens which then bind with antibody to form immune complexes.

Studies of the feasibility of screening people by means of faecal occult blood testing have shown that it is possible to detect asymptomatic cancers at an early stage. However, there are problems with these tests in the number of false-positives obtained due to dietary factors and also the levels of sensitivity needed to detect the maximum number of cancers and polyps. The use of immunological methods to test for tumour-related products in the faeces may hold out the greatest hope for screening studies in the future.

References

Aldercreutz H, Liewendahl K, Virkola P (1980) More on faecal occult blood testing. Gastroenterology 79: 959–960

Alm T, Licznerski G (1973) The intestinal polyposes. Clin Gastroenterol 2: 577–602

Bara J, Loisillier F, Burtin P (1980) Antigens of gastric and intestinal mucous cells in human colonic tumours. Br J Cancer 41: 209–221

Barrows GH, Burton RM, Jarrett DD, Russell GG, Alford D, Songster CL (1978) Immunochemical detection of human blood in faeces. Am J Clin Pathol 69: 342–346

Bassett ML, Goulston KJ (1980) False positive and negative Hemoccult reactions on a normal diet and effect of diet restriction. Aust NZ J Med 10: 1–4

Beretta KR, Guller R, Singeisen M, Stalder GA (1978) Occult blood in feces – a prospective study for comparison of Hemoccult and Fecatest. Schweiz Med Wochenschr 108: 1905–1907

Bohlman TW, Katon RM, Lipshutz GR, McCool MF, Smith FW, Melnyk CS (1977) Fiberoptic pansigmoidoscopy: An evaluation and comparison with rigid sigmoidoscopy. Gastroenterology 72: 644–649

Boyd JB, Bradford B, Watne AL (1980) Operative risk factors of colon resections in the elderly. Ann Surg 192: 743–746

Brahme F, Ekelund GR, Norden JR, Wackest A (1974) Metachronous colorectal polyps: comparison of development of colorectal polyps and carcinomas in persons with and without histories of polyps. Dis Colon Rectum 17: 166–171

Bralow SP (1979) Colorectal cancer screening program in Serasota, Florida. Symposium on Colorectal Cancer, New York

Brault J, Favre H (1979) Evaluation en pratique hospitalière du Fecatest, un nouvel examen de laboratoire pour la recherche de sang occulte dans les selles. Schweiz Med Wochenschr 109: 73–76

Bremner CG, Ackerman LV (1970) Polyps and carcinoma of the large bowel in the South African Bantu. Cancer 26: 991–999

Bussey HJR (1975) Familial polyposis coli. John Hopkins' University Press, Baltimore

Cameron AD (1960) Gastrointestinal blood loss measured by radioactive chromium. Gut 1: 177–182

Chester Beatty Research Institute, Harlow Industrial Health Service (1966) Precautions for laboratory workers who handle carcinogenic aromatic amines. Chester Beatty Research Institute, London

Clarke DN, Jones P, Needham CD (1980) Outcome in colorectal carcinoma: Seven-year study of a population. Br Med J 1: 431–435

Colin R, Le Grix A, Paillot B, Aubet JP, Cayron G, Robinson P, Metayer P, Geffroy Y (1978) Detection of polyps or cancers of the colon and rectum. The reliability of a test for fecal blood determination using platelets impregnated with guaiac. Nouv Presse Med 7: 1204–1205

Correa P, Strong JP, Reif A, Johnson WD (1977) Epidemiology of colorectal polyps. Cancer 39: 2258–2264

Doran J, Arden-Jones J, Hardcastle JD (to be published) Patterns of bleeding in colorectal cancer – the effect of aspirin. Implications for faecal occult blood testing. Br J Surg

Durst J, Neumann G, Schmidt K (1976) Okkultes Blut im Stuhl. Dtsch Med Wochenschr 101: 440–443

Ebaugh FC, Beeken WL (1959) Quantitative measurement of gastrointestinal blood loss. II. Determination of 24-hour fecal blood loss by a chemical photospectrometric technique. J Lab Clin Med 53: 777–788

Ebaugh FG, Clemens T, Rodnan G, Petersen RE (1958) Quantitative measurement of gastrointestinal blood loss. Am J Med 25: 169–181

Eide TJ, Stalsberg H (1978) Polyps of the large intestine in North Norway. Cancer 42: 2839–2848

Enterline HT (1974) Pathology of colonic polyps as it relates to surgical management. Ann Clin Lab Sci 4: 145–150

Falterman KW, Hill CB, Markey JC, Fox JW, Cohn I (1974) Cancer of the colon, rectum and anus: A review of 2313 cases. Cancer 34: 951–959

Farrands PA, Griffiths RL, Britton DC (1981) The Frome experiment: Value of screening for colorectal cancer. Lancet 1: 1231–1232

Fenoglio CM, Lane N (1974) The anatomical precursor of colorectal carcinoma. Cancer 34: 819–823

Filipe MI, Branfoot AC (1974) Abnormal patterns of mucus secretion in apparently normal mucosa of large intestine with carcinoma. Cancer 34: 282–290

Foster GE, Vellacott KD, Balfour TW, Hardcastle JD (1981) Outpatient flexible fiberoptic sigmoidoscopy, diagnostic yield and the value of glucagon. Br J Surg 68: 463–464

Freed DLJ, Taylor G (1972) Carcinoembryonic antigen in faeces. Br Med J 1: 85

Frühmorgen P, Demling L (1978) Erste Ergebnisse einer prospektiven Feldstudie mit einem modifizierten Guajak-Test zum Nachweis von okkultem Blut im Stuhl. In: Kolorektale Krebsvorsorge. Wachholz, Nürnberg, S 68–72

Fujimoto S, Kitsukawa U, Itoh K (1979) Carcinoembryonic antigen (CEA) in gastric juice or feces as an aid to diagnosis of gastrointestinal cancer. Ann Surg 189: 34–38

Gilbertsen VA (1974) Proctosigmoidoscopy and polypectomy in reducing the incidence of rectal cancer. Cancer 34: 936–939

Gilbertsen VA, Nelms JM (1978) The prevention of invasive cancer of the rectum. Cancer 41: 1137–1139

Gilbertsen VA, McHugh R, Schuman L, Williams SE (1980) The earlier detection of colorectal cancers. A preliminary report of the results of the occult blood study. Cancer 45: 2899–2901

Gill PG, Morris PJ (1978) The survival of patients with colorectal cancer treated at a regional hospital. Br J Surg 65: 17–20

Gillespie PE, Chambers TJ, Chan K, Doronzo F, Morson BC, Williams CB (1979) Colonic adenomas – a colonoscopy survey. Gut 20: 240–245

Glober GA, Peskoe SM (1974) Outpatient screening for gastrointestinal lesions using guaiac-impregnated slides. Dig Dis 19: 399–403

Gnauk R (1980) World Health Organization criteria for screening. In: Winawer SJ, Schottenfield D, Sherlock P (eds) Colorectal cancer: Prevention, epidemiology, and screening. Raven Press, New York, pp 175–180

Goldenberg DM, Kim EE, Deland FH, Bennett S, Primus FJ (1980) Radioimmunodetection of cancer with radioactive antibodies to carcinoembryonic antigen. Cancer Res 40: 2984–2992

Greaves P, Filipe MI, Branfoot AC (1980) Transitional mucosa and survival in human colorectal cancer. Cancer 46: 764–770

Greegor DH (1971) Occult blood testing for detection of asymptomatic colon cancer. Cancer 28: 131–134

Grossman ML, Matsumoto KK, Lichter RJ (1961) Fecal blood loss produced by oral and intravenous administration of various salicylates. Gastroenterology 40: 383–388

Hardcastle JD (1980) Screening for colorectal cancer. In: Wright R (ed) Recent advances in gastrointestinal pathology. Saunders, Philadelphia, pp 311–329

Hardcastle JD, Balfour TW, Amar SS (1980) Screening for symptomless colorectal cancer by testing for occult blood in general practice. Lancet 1: 791–793

Harvey JC (1956) The lack of effect of ingested ferrous sulphate on the guaiac test for occult blood in the stool. Am J Med Sci 232: 17–19

Hastings JB (1974) Mass screening for colorectal cancer. Am J Surg 127: 228–233

Helfrick GB, Petrucci P (1979) Public screening with fecal occult blood testing. Symposium on Colorectal Cancer, New York

Herzog P, Holtermüller K-H, Preiss J, Fischer J, Ewe K, Michaelis J (1981) Quantification of the intestinal blood loss in patients with colorectal polyps by 51-chromium-labeled erythrocytes and comparison with the Haemoccult test. Second International Symposium on Colorectal Cancer, Washington DC

Irons GV, Kirsner JB (1965) Routine chemical test of the stool for occult blood: An evaluation . Am J Med Sci 249: 247–260

Jaffe RM, Zierdt W (1979) A new occult blood test not subject to false negative results from reducing substances. J Lab Clin Med 93: 879–886

Jaffe RM, Kasten B, Young DS, Mallowry JD (1975) False negative stool occult blood test caused by ingestion of ascorbic acid (vitamin C). Ann Intern Med 83: 824–826

James WG (1977) Communication to a meeting of the American Society of Preventative Oncology, New York

Jones NCH (1958) Measurement of red-cell loss from gastrointestinal tract using radioactive chromium. Br Med J 1: 493–496

Jorge AD, Sanchez D, Diaz M, Lorenzo J, Milutin C (1977) Early detection of colonic and rectal cancer, extensive study of occult blood. Acta Gastroenterol Latinoam 7: 261–268

Katon RM, Lipshutz GR, McCool MF, Mayer B (1977) Fiberoptic sigmoidoscopy as a screening examination for retection of colonic neoplasia. Digestion 16: 250

Kawasaki H, Kimito E (1974) Mucosal glycoproteins in carcinoma cells of gastrointestinal tract, as detected by immunofluorescence technique. Acta Pathol Jpn 24: 481–494

Krasner N, Sumner D, Miller S, Thomson TJ, Goldberg A (1975) Assessment of Peroheme-40 for the presence of occult blood in faeces. Scott Med J 20: 329–332

Kuroki M, Koga Y, Matsuoka Y (1981) Purification and characterization of carcinoembryonic antigen-related antigens in normal adult faeces. Cancer Res 41: 713–720

Lipshutz GR, Katon RM, McCool MF, Mayer B, Smith FW, Duffy T, Melnyk CS (1979) Flexible sigmoidoscopy as a screening procedure for neoplasia of the colon. Surg Gynaecol Obstet 148: 19–22

Lockhart-Mummery HE, Ritchie JK, Hawley PR (1976) The results of surgical treatment for carcinoma of the rectum at St Mark's Hospital from 1948–1972. Br J Surg 63: 673–677

Mach J-P, Jaeger PH, Bertolet M-M, Ruegsegger C-H, Lossli RM, Pettavel J (1974) Detection of recurrence of large bowel carcinoma by radioimmunoassay of circulating C.E.A. Lancet 2: 535–540

Mach J-P, Carrel S, Forni M, Ritschard J, Donath A, Alberto P (1980) Tumour localisation of radiolabelled antibodies against carcinoembryonic antigens in patients with carcinoma. N Engl J Med 303: 5–10

Manier JW (1978) Fiberoptic pansigmoidoscopy: an evaluation of its use in an office practice. Gastrointest Endosc 24: 119–120

Marks G, Boggs W, Castro AF, Gathwright JB, Ray JE, Salvati E (1979) Sigmoidoscopic examinations with rigid and flexible fiberoptic sigmoidoscopes in the surgeons office: A comparative prospective study of effectiveness in 1,012 cases. Dis Colon Rectum 22: 162–168

Mayo CW, de Castro CA (1956) Carcinoma of the sigmoid arising from a polyp first visualised fifteen years previously: a report of case. Proc Mayo Clin 31: 597–598

Miller SF, Knight AR (1977) The early detection of colorectal cancer. Cancer 40: 945–949

Million R, Howarth J, Turnberg G, Turner LA (1980) Faecal occult blood screening in general practice. Gut 21: A921
Moertel CG, Hill JR, Docherty MB (1966) The routine proctoscopic examinations: a second look. Proc Mayo Clin 41: 368–374
Molnar IG, Vandevoorde JP, Gitnick GL (1976) C.E.A. levels in fluids bathing gastrointestinal tumours. Gastroenterology 70: 513–515
Morris DW, Hansell JR, Ostrow JD, Lee CS (1976) Reliability of chemical tests for fecal occult blood in hospitalised patients. Am J Dig Dis 21: 845–852
Morson BC (1966) Factors influencing the prognosis of early cancer of the rectum. Proc R Soc Med 59: 607–608
Morson BC (1974) The polyp-cancer sequence in the large bowel. Proc R Soc Med 67: 451–457
Morson BC (1976) Genesis of colorectal cancer. Clin Gastroenterol 5: 505–524
Needham CD, Simpson RG (1952) The benzidine test for occult blood in faeces. Q J Med 45: 123–133
Norfleet RG, Roberts RC (1979) Haemoccult screening for colorectal neoplasms: Report of a pilot study. Wis Med J 78: 25–27
Ostrow JD (1981) Attempts to improve detection of colon cancer with fecal occult blood tests. Second International Symposium on Colorectal Cancer, Washington DC
Ostrow JD, Mulvaney CA, Hansell JR, Rhodes RS (1973) Sensitivity and reproducibility of chemical tests for fecal occult blood with an emphasis on false positive reactions. Am J Dig Dis 18: 930–940
Otto P, Bunnemann H, Hans-Joachim X (1979) Screening and diagnosis in colorectal neoplasia. Symposium on Colorectal Cancer, New York
Parkins RA, Barrison IG (1981) The role of Haemoccult? Communication to the Workshop on Colorectal Cancer, London
Payne RA (1976) The incidence and clinical significance of rectal polyps. Ann R Coll Surg Engl 58: 241–242
Poleski MH, Blattner WA, Chatt H, Winawer SJ, Fleisher M, Schwartz MK, Fraumeni JF, Lipkin M (1978) C.E.A. in colonic lavage of individuals at high risk for large bowel cancer. Gastroenterology 74: 1140
Ransom MB, Shouler PJ, Tuley NJ, Hunt RH (1980) Does upper gastrointestinal bleeding affect the Haemoccult slide test for faecal occult blood? Br J Surg 67: 818
Ribet A, Frexinos J, Escourrou J, Delpu J (1980) Occult blood tests and colorectal tumours. Lancet 1: 417
Richardson JL (1977) Colorectal cancer: a mass screening and education programme. Geriatrics 123–131
Roche M, Perez-Gimmenez ME, Layrisse M, Diprisco E (1957) Study of urinary and fecal excretion of radioactive Cr^{51} in man: its use in the measurement of intestinal blood loss associated with hookworm infection. J Clin Invest 36: 1183–1192
Rogers GT, Keep PA (1980) C.E.A.-like activity in normal colon tissue. Eur J Cancer 16: 127–131
Rosenfield RE, Kochwa S, Kaczera Z, Maimon J (1979) Non-uniform distribution of occult blood in feces. Am J Clin Pathol 71: 204–209
Ross TH, Johnson JCM (1976) Detecting colorectal cancer. Ariz Med 33: 445–448
Rozen P, Fireman Z, Terdiman R, Hellerstein SM, Ratton J, Gilat T (1980) Selective screening for colorectal tumours in the Tel Aviv area: technique and initial results. In: Winawer SJ, Schottenfield D, Sherlock P (eds) Colorectal cancer: Presentation, epidemiology and screening. Raven Press, New York, pp 275–283
Samec HJ (1979) Haemoccult in colorectal carcinoma in Austria. Symposium on Colorectal Cancer, New York
Schwartz FW, Holstein H, Brecht JG (1980) Preliminary report on fecal occult blood testing in Germany. In: Winawer SJ, Schottenfield D, Sherlock P (eds) Colorectal cancer: Prevention, epidemiology, and screening. Raven Press, New York, pp 176–179

Sherlock S, Winawer SJ (1977) The role of early diagnosis in controlling large bowel cancer. Cancer (Suppl 5) 40: 2609–2615

Siba S (1980) Experience with Hemoccult screening in Hungary. (Multicentre studies) Orv Hetil 121: 1701–1703

Songster CL, Barrows GH, Jarrett DD (1980) Immunochemical detection of fecal occult blood – the fecal smear punch-disc test: a new non-invasive screening test for colorectal cancer. Cancer 45: 1099–1102

Spinelli P, Bertario L, Berrino F (1979) Guaiac test – our experience and evaluation program of efficacy. Symposium on Colorectal Cancer, New York

Stroehlein JR, Fairbanks VF, McGill DB, Go VLW (1976) Hemoccult detection of fecal occult blood quantitated by radioassay. Am J Dig Dis 21: 841–844

Thornton GHM, Illingworth G (1955) An evaluation of the benzidine test for occult blood in feces. Gastroenterology 28: 593–605

Till AS (1977) The results of treatment in district general hospitals. Topics in Gastroenterology 5: 77–85

Vellacott KD, Baldwin RW, Balfour TW, Hardcastle JD (1981a) Circulating immune complexes in patients with benign and malignant colorectal tumours. Br J Surg 68: 402–404

Vellacott KD, Baldwin RW, Hardcastle JD (1981b) An immunofluorescent test for faecal occult blood. Lancet 1: 18–19

Welch CE (1979) Polyps and cancer of the colon. Am J Surg 138: 625–626

Winawer SJ, Miller DG, Schottenfield D, Leidner SD, Sherlock P, Befler B, Stearns MW (1977) Feasibility of fecal occult blood testing for detection of colorectal neoplasia. Cancer 40: 2616–2619

Winawer SJ, Fleisher M, Green S, Bhargava D, Leidner SD, Boyle C, Sherlock P, Schwartz MK (1977b) C.E.A. in colonic lavage. Gastroenterology 73: 719–722

Winawer SJ, Andrews M, Flehinger B, Sherlock P, Schottenfield D, Miller DG (1980) Progress report on controlled trial of fecal occult blood testing for the detection of colorectal neoplasia. Cancer 45: 2959–2964

Winchester DP, Shull JH, Scanlon EF, Murrell JV, Smeltzer C, Vrba P, Iden M, Streelman DH, Magpayo R, Dow JW, Sylvester J (1980) A mass screening program for colorectal cancer using chemical testing for occult blood in the stool. Cancer 45: 2955–2958

Withers JN, James WC (1978) Colon cancer detection using guaiac screening. Hawaii Med J 37: 363–365

Wolff WI, Shinya H (1978) The impact of colonoscopy on the problem of colorectal cancer. Prog Clin Cancer 7: 51–69

Surgery

R. J. Nicholls

St. Mark's Hospital and St. Bartholomew's Hospital, London EC1V 2PS, United Kingdom

At present, surgery is the only form of treatment which offers a prospect of cure to patients with carcinoma of the colon. Although radiotherapy for carcinoma of the rectum holds some promise, surgery is still the treatment of choice for this disease also.

Pathological Factors

Over the last 30 years, survival after surgical removal of both rectal and colonic carcinomas has not changed. For example, at St. Mark's Hospital 40 out of every 100 patients with rectal cancer attending between 1948 and 1952 survived 5 years, as against 42 for the period 1968–1972. All other workers who have examined their results have found the same. This observation goes hand in hand with unchanging proportions of Dukes' stages A, B, and C over the same period. Thus, for rectal cancer the proportions at St. Mark's Hospital of A, B, and C lesions of 15%, 33%, and 52% during the quinquennium 1948–1952 are not significantly different from 15%, 41%, and 44% during 1968–1972. Again, similar observations have been made by all who have reported their results for rectal or colonic carcinoma over these years. It is apparent that the pathology of the tumour is the most important determinant of the results of surgery. Pathological features influencing survival include not only the Dukes' stage and histological grade, but also the presence of invasion by tumour of nearby veins and the degree of direct local spread of the tumour outside the rectal wall. The last two features have received less attention than they deserve. The effect on survival of these factors among patients having radical or curative, resection for rectal cancer is demonstrated in Table 1. There is a notable fall in survival with lymph node involvement or extramural venous invasion, when direct local spread is extensive, and when the tumour is of a high grade of malignancy (anaplastic).

The reported results of surgery vary, however. As shown in Fig. 1 the 5-year survival rate among five surgical series selected for the large number of patients ranged from 28% in the Birmingham region (Slaney 1951) to over 50% in Leeds (Whittaker and Goligher 1976) and at St. Mark's Hospital (Lockhart Mummery et al. 1976). The reason for this disparity must be largely due to the proportion of patients in whom it was possible to carry out a radical operation. It can be seen in Fig. 1 that there is a close linear relationship between this variable and survival.

The proportion of patients having radical operations is determined by the pathological stage of the tumour, and differences in the degree of advancement largely explain the differences in survival rates reported. Among patients presenting to the United

Recent Results in Cancer Research, Vol. 83

Table 1. Influence of pathological factors on survival (corrected 5-year survival as percentage) following radical removal

	Dukes' stage		Histological grade
A	92.5	Low	76.5
B	77.0	Average	78.0
C	30.5	High	59.0
	Venous invasion		Degree of extrarectal spread
Absent	71.0	Slight	75.0
Present	42.0	Moderate	57.0
		Extensive	27.0

From Dukes' and Bussey 1958; Talbot et al. 1980

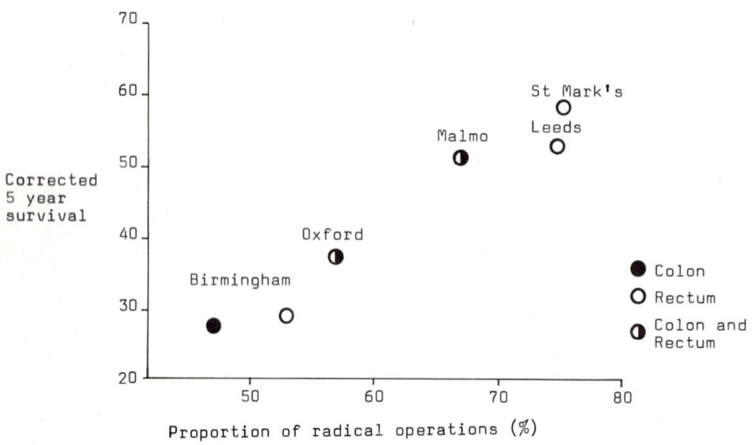

Fig. 1. Relationship of proportion of radical operations and survival among all patients seen with large-bowel cancer at various centres

Oxford Hospitals between 1966 and 1971, only about 6% had Dukes' A tumours and nearly one-third (30.4%) already had distant metastases (Gill and Morris 1978). In contrast, at St. Mark's Hospital over a similar period 11% of all patients attending had Dukes' A tumours and only about 10% presented with disseminated disease. These different distributions of pathological stage can be explained largely by differences in the number of patients admitted as emergencies with obstruction or perforation. Such patients account for about 40% of all admissions for large-bowel cancer to a district general hospital, in contrast to less than 5% of admissions to a specialist centre. Nearly half these patients have metastases on presentation and, furthermore, there is a high proportion of Dukes' C cases among those without dissemination. The hospital mortality of this group of seriously ill and often old patients is around 20%–30%, adding further to the poor outlook (Till 1977).

Surgical Factors

Although the pathology of the tumour is the chief determinant of the results of surgery, it is important to consider whether there are any surgical factors per se which can influence survival. Does the resectability rate depend upon a variation among surgeons in their alacrity to remove the primary tumour as well as on pathological factors? If there is such a variation, does this affect the results? Is the extent of resection, for example, the size of the field of lymph node removal or mesentery excised likely to improve survival? Is the 'no-touch' isolation technique of benefit?

Resectability Rate

Peloquin (1973) analysed the results obtained by 21 surgeons treating patients with large bowel cancer seen at a single hospital over a 24-year period. The surgeons were divided into three groups 'conservative', 'intermediate', and 'aggressive'. This somewhat subjective division was made on the basis of the extent of resection they normally carried out, judged by the amount of contiguous bowel and mesentery excised and the willingness to remove other locally invaded structures. When the results of the conservative and aggressive surgeons were compared, a significant difference in the resectability rate was found. The former group removed the primary tumour in 72% of patients, as against 92% removed by the latter. This difference could be explained by a higher proportion of locally advanced growths presenting to the conservative surgeons, but the survival rates obtained by each group suggest that a surgeon-related difference was more likely to be responsible. The overall 5-year survival of 248 patients treated by the conservative surgeons was 35%, in contrast to 47% of 323 patients treated by the aggressive surgeons. This difference was almost completely accounted for by the difference in the number of patients whose cancer was not resected. The survival of patients with resected growths was around 40% whether treated by the conservative or the aggressive surgeons. Thus, an improved survival rate can be obtained by increasing the resectability rate. The surgeon should do his best, therefore, to remove the primary tumour wherever possible.

Mesenteric Clearance

It is important to consider whether the extent of excision of the lymphovascular field draining the tumour can influence survival. It is feasible to divide the main artery and vein of the segment of bowel to be removed at their points of origin with no apparently increased hazard for the patient. There is little information to date on this question. A recent retrospective study among patients undergoing resections for cancer of the rectum and rectosigmoid junction indicates that ligation of the inferior mesenteric artery at its origin from the aorta may be of value (R. J. Nicholls, 1981, unpublished work). The records of all patients undergoing radical resections at St. Mark's Hospital between 1958 and 1972 were studied. During that time four of the eight staff surgeons usually ligated the inferior mesenteric artery flush with the aorta (high ligation), while the other four surgeons usually made their ligation distal to the origin of the left colic artery (low ligation), with corresponding levels of ligation of the inferior mesenteric vein. The patients were divided into 'high' and 'low' ligation groups, and the 5-year survival rates for tumours of similar pathological stages were compared. The distribution of histological grades of tumours was similar in each group. No difference in survival for patients with Dukes' A, B, or C_2 tumours was found; in the case of patients with Dukes' C_1 tumours and fewer than five lymph nodes involved there was a significant difference when the growth was sited in the middle or upper rectum or at the rectosigmoid junction. The corrected 5-year survival rate in 114 patients after high ligation was 65.5%, as against 46.7% in 88 patients who underwent a low ligation for tumours in this category ($\chi^2 = 6.1$, $P < 0.01$). While it is recognized that this is not a controlled study these data suggest that a more extensive mesenteric clearance may possible improve the survival of some patients.

Extended Lymphadenectomy

Pelvic lymphadenectomy is a good example of an extended lymphatic removal and is practised widely throughout the world although little in the United Kingdom. It is carried out for rectal cancer in combination with excision of the primary tumour. The rationale for this manoeuvre is the knowledge that lymphatic and venous spread of rectal carcinomas below the peritoneal reflection occurs not only upwards along the inferior mesenteric pedicle but also laterally to the lateral pelvic wall via the middle rectal vessels and lymphatics. Sauer and Bacon (1952) found involved lateral pelvic lymph nodes in 6 of 21 patients with extraperitoneal rectal cancer and advocated pelvic lymphadenectomy as a result of this observation. Stearns and Deddish (1959) have reported the largest series of patients treated by pelvic lymphadenectomy in addition to resection of the rectum. Only 11 (9%) of 122 patients had microscopically confirmed spread to the pelvic nodes. There was a high complication rate, with permanent neurogenic bladder dysfunction being particularly common. The operation cannot be justified from these results.

No Touch Technique

This method of surgical excision was advocated by Turnbull of the Cleveland Clinic, based on the hypothesis that mobilization of the tumour by the surgeon causes tumour cells to be liberated into the circulation, which may then lodge in distant sites to develop into metastases. It involves ligation of the arterial supply and venous drainage of the segment of bowel to be resected before mobilization of the tumour. Turnbull et al. (1967) reported a crude 5-year survival rate of 69% among 460 patients having a radical resection for carcinoma of the colon. The 5-year survival rate of 58% for Dukes' C lesions appeared to be higher than the results obtained by other surgeons at the time. However, in two subsequent comparable series at Memorial Hospital, New York (Stearns and Schottenfeld 1971) and St. Mark's Hospital (J. K. Ritchie, 1981, unpublished work) the overall crude survival rates were 69% and 66%, and those for Dukes' C tumours were 52% and 54%. It seems unlikely, therefore, that the no touch technique influences survival.

Advances in Surgery

There have been several advances in the surgical management of large-bowel cancer during the last 10–20 years. The operative mortality has been reduced owing to improvements in anaesthesia and pre- and postoperative care. At St. Mark's Hospital, the operative mortality fell from about 9% in 1950 to 2.5% in 1972. In addition, the use of prophylactic antibiotics given around the time of operation has reduced the incidence of postoperative wound infections and new methods of bowel preparation, such as whole-gut irrigation, have been introduced. Surgery has been applied more generally to the treatment of advanced disease, whether distant metastases or local recurrence, partly as a result of improved diagnostic techniques for the detection and assessment of these lesions.

The outstanding advance has been the increasing application of sphincter-preserving operations, as either a major resection or a local treatment for rectal cancer. In contrast, there has been little change in the surgical technique for treating carcinoma of the colon. During the last 30 years there has been a marked trend away from total rectal excision in favour of restorative resection. At St. Mark's Hospital 85% of patients with rectal cancer were treated by total rectal excision in the 1950s, whereas by 1975 this had fallen to 45% (Fig. 2). The majority, therefore, are now treated by major restorative resection or local excision. Although one would like to see the proportion of sphincter-preserving operations rise still further, it is likely that the curves will now tend to become horizontal, since the indications for restorative procedures are limited by the pathology and site of the tumour.

The chief reason for this trend has been the increasing application of restorative operations for cancers of the middle rectum. These tumours lie from about 12 cm down to 7 or 8 cm from the anal verge. It should be appreciated that the lowest tumours in this region are at most only about 3–4 cm above the anal verge, since the anal canal is about 4 cm in length. Pathological studies investigating the extent of spread of microscopic tumour distal to the cancer indicate that such spread for a distance greater than 1.5 cm is rare, occurring in less than 5% of cases (Quer et al. 1953; Penfold 1974). It seems, therefore, that a major resection taking a 3-cm length of bowel below the tumour would adequately remove any distal spread in most cases. The chance of distal spread for a greater distance is increased when the tumour is

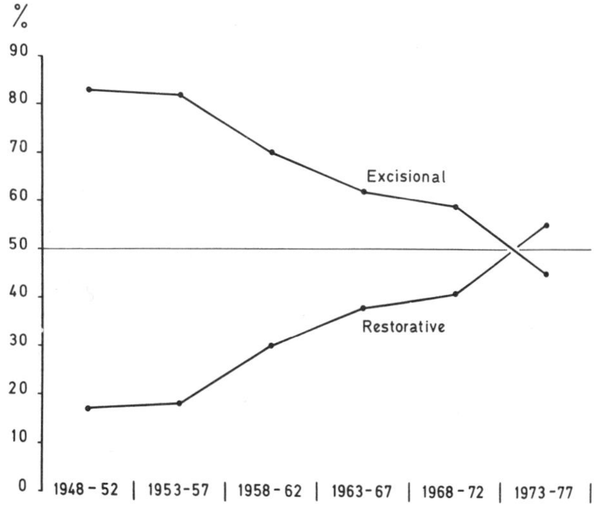

Fig. 2. Type of surgery performed for carcinoma of the rectum in St. Mark's Hospital, 1948–1977

anaplastic. For this reason many surgeons have been reluctant to carry out restorative resections for such cancers at this level. However, a recent study suggests that survival after restorative resection or total rectal excision of anaplastic carcinoma of the middle rectum is no different (Elliot and Nicholls 1980). A large cancer in the middle rectum which the surgeon considers is likely to recur locally, for example if it is not certain that removal has been complete, should be treated by a total rectal excision. This avoids the problem of persistent or recurrent tumour in the vicinity of an anastomosis. It may also be inadvisable to carry out a major restorative resection involving a very distal anastomosis in a patient with distant metastases. Recovery of bowel function postoperatively following the initial delay in closure of a temporary colostomy may take several months of the patient's short life expectancy.

It is important to know whether major restorative resections for middle-third carcinomas are as curative as total rectal excision. Five-year survival rates after either operation for middle rectal cancers of similar Dukes' stage and histological grade were found to be similar in a retrospective study of patients subjected to radical major surgery.

Those with Dukes' B tumours of average grade had 5-year survival rates of 61% and 69%, respectively, after anterior resection and total rectal excision.

Major Restorative Operations

There are several techniques available for carrying out a major sphincter-preserving operation for carcinoma of the rectum. They differ in the method of anastomosis employed, but not in the extent of abdominal dissection. Anterior resection is the commonest of these operations. It is divided into high anterior resection, where the anastomosis is made per abdomen above the level of the peritoneal reflection, and low anterior resection, where it is made below. Other methods of constructing colorectal or coloanal anastomosis include the peranal technique (Parks 1972), pull-through procedures (Bacon 1945; Turnbull and Cuthbertson 1961; Cutait and Figlioni 1961), and abdominosacral operations (Localio et al. 1978; York Mason 1972).

Anterior Resection

The cardinal complication of large-bowel surgery is anastomotic leakage, and this accounts for one-third to one-half of postoperative deaths (Vandertoll and Beahrs 1965). There is considerable variation in the reported rate of leakage, from less than 5% to as high as 30%, and there is some evidence to indicate that the complication may be surgeon-related (Fielding et al. 1978). Direct aetiological factors include tension, poor blood supply of the bowel, and local haematoma and abscess formation draining postoperatively into the bowel lumen via the anastomosis. The anastomotic leakage rate is highest for low anterior resection, being of the order of 10%–20% judging by pelvic abscess or faecal fistula formation. A considerably higher rate of subclinical leakage is determined by radiological examination.

In the last 5 years mechanical stapling devices have been used increasingly in large-bowel surgery. Although it should be pointed out that such instruments have been in existence for many years, it is only recently that they have been used to construct colorectal and coloanal anastomoses. This has become possible with the development of the circular stapling device, initially in Russia (Fain et al. 1975). The use of this instrument has raised two questions, first, whether more restorative operations are now possible, and secondly, whether the rate of leakage is lower than with conventional hand suturing. In answer to the first, there is already evidence that the number of total rectal excisions is being reduced (Heald 1980). The reason for this is not, as the general public may have gathered, that the stapling gun enables anastomoses where none could be made before; the other techniques mentioned above have been in existence for many years and it is possible to use these to make an anastomosis in almost all cases. The more likely reason is that the gun is an attractive proposition to surgeons who do not use these other methods, as it enables a low anterior resection to be made more easily than is often the case with hand suturing. The question as to whether the rate of leakage is reduced cannot be answered at the moment. Goligher et al. (1979) reported clinical leakage in two out of 62 patients having a stapled anastomosis. These included 24 low anterior resections, a rate considerably lower than their previous experience with hand suturing. Higher rates with stapling, around 10%, have been reported by others (Heald 1980), however, but controlled clinical trials are required. A preliminary report of a trial comparing stapled and hand-sutured (both one- and two-layer) anastomoses, suggests there is little difference between these methods (Overy et al. 1980), but further results are awaited.

Coloanal Anastomosis

This operation was developed by Parks (1972) and enables an anastomosis between the colon and anal canal to be made by means of a per anal suturing technique. The patient is placed in the Trendelenberg position with the legs raised and everted on crutches. The rectum with the growth is mobilized per abdomen and a bowel clamp is applied below the tumour. The rectum is divided below the clamp and the specimen removed. The surgeon then takes up a position facing the perineum and passes a self-retaining retractor into the anus. The colon is delivered per anum from above into the perineal field and joined to the anal or short rectal stump by interrupted absorbable (Dexon) sutures. A modification of this technique is now preferred, whereby the mucosa from the distal stump is removed down to the dentate line and the anastomosis is then carried out at this level. In this way a short cuff or sleeve of upper anal canal and lower rectal musculature envelops the last 2–3 cm of colon with the aim of offering protection against dehiscence.

This operation has been carried out in 76 patients with an operative mortality of 2.6%. In 17% there was some degree of pelvic sepsis, usually considered minor. Rectal continence postoperatively was normal in 50% of patients and almost normal with disturbances of holding flatus in a further 45%. Too few patients have been followed long enough for 5-year survival rates to be known, but the crude 3-year survival rate of all patients having radical operations was 69%. Local recurrence has occurred in 10% of all patients undergoing either palliative or radical resection.

Pull-Through Procedures

There are several modifications of this operation, but all have a common basic principle. After removal of the operative specimen the colon is passed through the anus to protrude for a distance of several centimetres. The patient is returned to the ward and a week to 10 days is allowed for adhesions between it and the distal anorectal stump to form. The redundant colon is then excised. In one modification, a direct suture between the trimmed colonic margin and the everted anorectum is carried out at this stage and the anastomosis allowed to retract spontaneously into the pelvis over the next few days. Bennett (1976) analysed the results of this operation reported from several centres. Operative mortality ranged from 2% to 12%, and approximately 80% of patients had normal or 'acceptable' continence. In some reports normal continence has been observed in only 30% of patients, suggesting that function after pull-through procedures is less satisfactory than after the peranal method of anastomosis. Five-year survival rates were 50%–60% after radical operations.

Abdominosacral Procedures

Approaches to the rectum described at the end of the last century have been modified most recently by Localio et al. (1978) and York Mason (1972). An abdominal dissection is combined with a sacral approach in both these versions. With Localio's method, the patient lies in the right lateral position and the specimen is removed per abdomen. A perineal operator enters the postrectal space through a transverse incision over the sacrum, removing the coccyx, and the anastomosis is made after delivery of the colon and distal rectal stump through the wound. In York Mason's transsphincteric modification, access to the postrectal space is gained by dividing the anal sphincters posteriorly, repairing them after the anastomosis has been made. Localio et al. (1978) reported an operative mortality of 2% among 100 patients treated. The 5-year survival rate after radical treatment was 58% and there were local recurrences in 17%. Normal continence was achieved in all patients.

Local Treatment

Local treatment has become of interest to surgeons and radiotherapists in recent years. Although total excision is the treatment of choice for most carcinomas of the lower rectum, a few may be curable by some form of local treatment. There are various methods including surgical excision, electrofulguration (Maden and Kandalaft 1971; Crile and Turnbull 1972), laser destruction, and contact radiotherapy (Papillon 1975). For the surgeon, excision is the favoured method and has the advantage over the other techniques that a specimen is available for pathological examination.

The difficulty of treating patients by local excision lies not in the execution of the method, but in the selection of patients. Local excision must remove the tumour entirely. It follows that where there is a high chance of lymph node metastases or of local recurrence later because of the extent of local spread, local excision is contraindicated. Suitable cancers are therefore small in diameter and confined to the rectum. They should not have lymph node metastases and must not be anaplastic. At present, the first three of these criteria can only be determined by digital examination of the tumour pre-operatively. It has been found that about 70% of tumours confined to the rectum can be recognized as such by this method. Enlarged retrorectal lymph nodes can be palpated in 50% of patients found subsequently by the pathologist to have lymph node involvement (R. J. Nicholls et al. 1981, unpublished work). Many surgeons would only consider local excision of ulcerating carcinomas in old patients who are unfit for major surgery, and would use a major restorative operation when the cancer lies sufficiently far above the anal sphincter for this to be possible.

The lower rectum can be readily approached via the anal canal with an anal retractor, but some prefer the transsphincteric exposure. The growth is circumcised at a distance of about 1 cm from its edge and removed with a full-thickness disc of rectal wall. The resulting wound is then sutured. The specimen should be pinned flat onto a cork board and fixed in that position to facilitate pathological examination. The policy of local excision is conditional upon the pathological findings. Thus evidence of penetration of the bowel wall or invasion of veins or lymphatics in the excised specimen is an indication for immediate major resection.

A series of 22 patients with ulcerating sessile carcinomas of the rectum treated by local excision were followed-up for 5 years. Fourteen patients required no further operation. Six patients were operated upon again as a result of the pathologist's report, two of whom had lymph node metastases, and two had subsequent rectal excision for local recurrences. Of the 22, there were 20 alive at 5 years (Lock et al. 1978), and it appears that provided patients are carefully selected there is a good prospect of long-term survival.

Management of Disseminated Disease

Some patients with disseminated disease are suitable for surgical resection of metastases with a prospect of prolonged survival. They appear to be those with solitary lesions in the liver or lung, although some with multiple metastases confined to one hepatic lobe may also be benefited. Unfortunately such patients are uncommon, comprising 5%–10% of those with liver metastases (Wood et al. 1976). Nevertheless, in this group there is some evidence that major hepatic resection may improve the outlook. Thus Adson and Van Heerden (1980) reported a 3-year survival rate of 41% of those among 32 patients surviving hepatic lobectomy who had been monitored for this time. This group included some with simultaneous metastases elsewhere or with multiple unilobar hepatic metastases. The 3-year survival rate of patients with apparently solitary metastases in the liver was around 50%. Similarly, 5-year survival rates of around 20% after resection of solitary lung metastases have been reported (McCormick and Attiyeh 1979).

Management of Local Recurrence

Although most miserable for the patient, especially if it occurs in the pelvis, local recurrence is not the cause of death in many patients. Berge et al. (1972) reported the results of a large series of autopsies on patients who had been treated for large-bowel cancer. The strength of their study was the high autopsy rate of 81% within the community under observation, and the results must be regarded as among the most accurate available on the distribution of tumour at death. It was found that of 267 patients autopsied who had had radical surgery, 207 had recurrent tumour, and 110 of these were found to have local recurrence. However, only 12 of the 110 patients had local recurrence without co-existing distant metastases.

It seems, therefore, that the resection of local recurrence, even if it is possible, is unlikely to cure the patient, and the results of surgery support this. Reported survival rates after apparently complete excision of local recurrence are about 5%–10% at 5 years. Since resection of tumour is possible in only 10%–20% of patients with local recurrence, however, the patients benefited are only a small fraction of the total. In an attempt to identify local recurrence at a stage where it would still be resectable, Wangensteen advocated a routine laparotomy some 6–12 months after the primary resection. He claimed that such 'second-look' procedures made it possible to remove 20% of local recurrences with a low mortality (Gilbertsen and Wangensteen 1962). This policy was not adopted by others, who considered that the disadvantages of postoperative complications, deaths, and poor survival rates outweighed the advantage of extending life for a small number of patients. It might be, however, that frequent monitoring of serum carcinoembryonic antigen (CEA) levels postoperatively may improve the resectability rate. It is clear that recurrence can be detected by this means, often with a so-called lead time over clinical detection of several months (Sorokin et al. 1974). Perhaps exploration at an earlier stage might reveal more resectable recurrences. Martin et al. (1979) reported a resectability rate of 70% when the decision for surgery was taken on rising CEA values alone, but the number of patients in this report was small.

Conclusions

The first aim of surgery in large-bowel cancer is to cure the disease with as little mortality and morbidity as possible. Cure will be more likely if the primary tumour is resected whenever possible, and it is therefore worthwhile including the resection of locally invaded organs to obtain local clearance. There is some evidence that the extent of mesenteric clearance is important for survival, but little is gained by extensive pelvic lymphatic removal in rectal carcinoma. There is every indication that sphincter-preserving operations (including local excision) for correctly selected tumours are as likely as total rectal excision to result in long-term survival. Surgery for metastatic disease or local recurrence results in a certain number of long-term survivors, but these form only a small proportion of the total number of patients with advanced disease.

References

Adson MA, Van Heerden JA (1980) Major hepatic resections for metastatic colo-rectal cancer. Ann Surg 191: 576–579

Bacon HE (1945) Evolution of sphincter muscle preservation and re-establishment of continuity in the operative treatment of rectal and sigmoidal cancer. Surg Gynaecol Obstet 81: 113–118

Bennet RC (1976) The place of pull-through operations in the treatment of carcinoma of the rectum. Dis Colon Rectum 19: 420–423

Berge T, Ekeland G, Mellner C, Wenckert P (1972) Carcinoma of the colon and rectum in a defined population. Acta Chir Scand [Suppl 438]

Crile G, Turnbull RB (1972) The role of electro-coagulation in the treatment of carcinoma of the rectum. Surg Gynaecol Obstet 135: 391–392

Cutait DE, Figlioni FJ (1961) A new method of colo-rectal anastomosis in abdomino-perineal resection. Dis Colon Rectum 4: 335–338

Dukes CE, Bussey HJR (1958) The spread of rectal cancer and its effect on prognosis. Br J Cancer 12: 309–313
Elliot ME, Nicholls RJ (1980) Radical surgery for high grade tumours of the mid-rectum. Gut 21: A902–905
Fain SN, Patin CS, Morgenstern L (1975) Use of a mechanical suturing apparatus in low colo-rectal anastomosis. Arch Surg 110: 1079–1082
Fielding LP, Stewart-Brown S, Dudley HAF (1978) Surgeon-related variables and the clinical trial. Lancet 2: 778–781
Gilbertsen VA, Wangensteen OH (1962) A summary of thirteen years' experience with the second-look program. Surg Gynaecol Obstet 114: 438–442
Gill PG, Morris PJ (1978) The survival of patients with colo-rectal cancer treated in a regional hospital. Br J Surg 65: 17–21
Goligher JC, Lee PWR, Macfie J, Simpkins KC, Lintott DJ (1979) Experience with the Russian model 249 suture gun for anastomosis of the rectum. Surg Gynaecol Obstet 148: 517–520
Heald RJ (1980) Towards fewer colostomies – the impact of circular stapling devices on the surgery of rectal cancer in a district hospital. Br J Surg 67: 198–200
Localio AS, Eng K, Gouge TH, Ranson JHC (1978) Abdomino-sacral resection for carcinoma of the mid rectum – ten years experience. An Surg 188: 475–479
Lock MR, Cairns DW, Ritchie JK, Lockhart Mummery HE (1978) The treatment of early colo-rectal cancer by local excision. Br J Surg 65: 346–351
Lockhart Mummery HE, Ritchie JK, Hawley PR (1976) The results of surgical treatment for carcinoma of the rectum at St Mark's Hospital from 1948 to 1972. Br J Surg 63: 673–678
Madden JL, Kandalaft S (1971) Clinical evaluation of electro-coagulation in the treatment of cancer of the rectum. Am J Surg 122: 347–351
Martin EW, Cooperman M, King G, Rinker L, Carey LC, Minton JP (1979 A retrospective and prospective study of social CEA determinations in the early detection of recurrent colon cancer. Am J Surg 137: 167–169
McCormack PM, Attiyah FF (1979) Resected pulmonary metastases from colo-rectal cancer. Dis Colon Rectum 22: 553–556
Overy RD, Godfrey PJ, Evans M, Pollock AV (1980) Staples or sutures in the colon? A random controlled trial of three methods of colonic anastomosis. Br J Surg 67: 363–368
Papillon J (1975) Intracavitary irradiation of early rectal cancer for cure. Cancer 36: 696–701
Parks AG (1972) Transanal technique in low rectal anastomosis. Proc R Scot Med 65: 975–979
Peloquin AB (1973) Cancer of the colon and rectum: Comparison of the results of three different groups of surgeons using different techniques. Can J Surg 16: 28–31
Penfold JCB (1974) A comparison of restorative resection of carcinoma of the middle-third of the rectum with abdomino-perineal excision. Aust NZ J Surg 44: 354–359
Quer EA, Dahlin DC, Mayo CW (1953) Retrograde intramural spread of carcinoma of the rectum and recto-sigmoid: a microscopic study. Surg Gynaecol Obstet 96: 24–27
Sauer I, Bacon HE (1952) A new approach for excision of carcinoma of the lower portion of the rectum and anal canal. Surg Gynaecol Obstet 95: 229–235
Slaney G (1971) Results of treatment of carcinoma of the colon and rectum. In: Irvine WT (ed) Modern trends in surgery, 3rd edn. Butterworths, London, pp 69–78
Sokorin JJ, Sugarbaker PH, Zamcheck N, Pisick M, Kupchik HZ, Moore FD (1974) Serial carcino-embryonic antigen assays. Use in detection of cancer recurrence. JAMA 228: 49–54
Stearns MW, Deddish MR (1959) Five-year results of abdomino-pelvic lymph node dissection for carcinom of the rectum. Dis Colon Rectum 2: 169–176
Stearns MW, Schottenfeld D (1971) Techniques for the surgical management of colon cancer. Cancer 28: 165–171

Talbot IC, Ritchie S, Leighton MH, Hughes AD, Bussey HJR, Morson BC (1980) The clinical significance of invasion of veins by rectal cancer. Br J Surg 67: 439–442

Till AS (1977) Cancer of the large bowel: The results of treatment in district general hospital. Topics in Gastroenterology 5: 77–84

Turnbull RB, Cuthbertson AM (1961) Abdomino-rectal pull-through resection of cancer and for Hirschsprung's disease. Cleve Clin Q 28: 109–112

Turnbull RB, Kyle K, Watson FR, Spratt J (1967) Cancer of the colon: The influence of the no-touch isolation technique on survival rates. Ann Surg 166: 420–422

Vandertoll DJ, Beahrs OH (1965) Carcinoma of rectum and low sigmoid. Evaluation of anterior resection of 1766 favourable lesions. Arch Surg 90: 793–796

Whittaker M, Goligher JC (1976) The prognosis after surgical treatment for carcinoma of the rectum. Br J Surg 63: 384–387

Wood CB, Gillis CR, Blumgart LH (1976) A retrospective study of the natural history of patients with liver metastases from colo-rectal cancer. Clin Oncol 2: 285–289

York Mason A (1972) Trans-sphincteric exposure for low rectal anastomosis. Proc R Soc Med 65: 974–977

Radiotherapy

S. J. Arnott

Department of Clinical Oncology, Western General Hospital, University of Edinburgh, Edinburgh EH4 2XU, United Kingdom

There has been a considerable change in attitude in recent years towards the use of radiotherapy in rectal cancer. This had come about partly because of an appreciation of the palliative value of x-ray therapy in patients with symptoms from inoperable or recurrent cancer, but also as a result of a greater awareness of the contribution irradiation may make to improved cure rates in early tumours.

Adenocarcinoma of the large bowel has traditionally been regarded as being a radioresistant tumour totally unsuited to management by radiotherapy. This is an attitude which developed during the days of low-energy orthovoltage equipment with which it was virtually impossible to deliver curative doses of irradiation to deep-seated tumours in the pelvis without at the same time delivering unacceptable high doses to normal tissues, particularly the small and large bowel. It was not until the advent of high-energy megavoltage radiotherapy equipment that the use of irradiation in the treatment of large-bowel cancer began to be fully explored. One of the first reports describing the effectiveness of radiotherapy in the relief of symptoms from advanced disease came from St. Bartholomew's Hospital in the 1950s (Williams and Horwitz 1956).

Patients were referred for consideration of radiotherapy if they were found to have inoperable disease resulting from tumour extent. However, a few patients were given treatment if poor general health prevented operation. The principal symptoms of pain, tenesmus, and discharge were completely relieved in about half the patients, with a further quarter obtaining partial relief. Bleeding was particularly effectively alleviated by this therapy. Interestingly, in this group of patients treatment resulted in a small 5-year survival of 5% (Table 1).

Combined Radiotherapy and Chemotherapy

Nevertheless, in spite of the encouraging results of this early work, there was little enthusiasm for the use of radiotherapy in rectal cancer until the 1960s, when work began on the investigation of combined treatment with chemotherapy and irradiation. The idea behind this was that the chemotherapy would enhance the effectiveness of radiotherapy. The concept of combined therapy was largely based on work carried out by Heidelberger and his group, who gave the drug 5-fluorouracil combined with x-rays (Heidelberger et al. 1958). These experiments demonstrated that when animals were given both x-ray treatment and a dose of 5-fluorouracil this combination was more effective than either radiotherapy or the drug itself in the control of growth of a variety of tumours. About this time it was realized that 5-fluorouracil was particularly

Recent Results in Cancer Research, Vol. 83

Table 1. Effectiveness of radiotherapy in relief of symptoms in rectal cancer

Symptom	No. of cases	Complete relief	Partial relief	Failure
Pain	102	49 (48%)	29 (29%)	24 (23%)
Tenesmus	66	36 (55%)	12 (18%)	18 (27%)
Discharge	116	47 (41%)	30 (26%)	39 (33%)
Bleeding	135	103 (76%)	18 (14%)	14 (10%)

From Williams and Horwitz (1956)

effective against large bowel cancer, and clinical work then began in a number of centres of evaluate the use of this combined regimen in patients with inoperable large bowel cancer. Whilst the concept of using a combination of drug therapy and radiation in the treatment of human tumours is attractive, it remains controversial therapy. Whilst some studies have indicated an improvement in results from combined regimens over those obtained with the use of radiotherapy alone, other workers have argued that it might have been possible to attain the same improvement in results by giving a higher dose of radiotherapy. Whilst the mechanism of interaction has not yet been fully elucidated, it is generally felt that for most human tumours radiation and cytotoxic drugs act in an additive fashion rather than a truly synergistic manner.
One of the first reports describing the effectiveness of combined radiation and chemotherapy in large-bowel cancer came from the Mayo clinic in the United States of America (Moertal et al. 1969). This demonstrated that both survival and symptomatic relief were improved in patients with unresectable carcinoma of the colon and rectum when they were treated with a combined regimen of 5-fluorouracil and radiotherapy. However, criticism has been levelled against this study, and in particular against the dose of radiation used, which was only of the order of 35 to 40 gray over a period of 4–4 $^1/_2$ weeks, and it has been argued that a similar improvement could have been achieved if the dose of radiation had been raised, rather than adding 5-fluorouracil to the treatment regimen. Other criticisms were that the method of giving 5-fluorouracil only during the first 3 days of radiotherapy was not optimal. Experimental evidence has suggested that it might be more effective if the 5-fluorouracil were given throughout the course of radiotherapy (Vietti et al. 1971).

Edinburgh Experience

Considerable experience of treating patients with inoperable and recurrent large bowel cancer has been gained in Edinburgh. Since 1968 a series of studies have been conducted on these patients in an attempt to evaluate the place of radiotherapy in their treatment.
Initially, patients were treated with a combined regimen of 5-fluorouracil and radiotherapy, but more recently radiotherapy alone has been used (Arnott 1975). A total of 325 patients has been evaluated to assess the effectiveness of radiotherapy. These are all unselected, consecutive patients referred to the Department of Radiotherapy with symptoms of inoperable or locally recurrent rectal cancer. All were deemed clinically to have inoperable or recurrent disease, and patients who refused surgery or were deemed inoperable on medical grounds have been excluded from this analysis.

Table 2. Results of palliative treatment (radiotherapy for inoperable tumours) of rectal cancer

Symptom	Complete response	Partial response	Failure
Pain	44.5%	29.6%	25.9%
Discharge	24.2%	37.9%	37.9%
Tumour	9.7%	58.0%	32.3%

Table 3. Results of palliative treatment (radiotherapy for recurrent disease) of recurrent disease in rectal cancer

Symptom	Complete response	Partial response	Failure
Pain	33.3%	40.0%	26.7%
Discharge	40.0%	10.0%	50.0%
Tumour	12.5%	54.2%	33.3%

As might be expected in such a group of patients, two-thirds were considered suitable to receive only palliative treatment and one-third received a more aggressive treatment.

Palliative Radiotherapy

Although the majority of the patients received only palliative radiotherapy, the symptomatic relief achieved was impressive. For example, most of those with inoperable cancers gained significant relief of pain and mucoid rectal discharge. The complete eradication of local tumour masses, however, was achieved in only a few patients. This is not particularly surprising, considering that many patients had enormous rectal tumours (Table 2).
Similar results were seen in patients treated palliatively for recurrent disease. Again, over half the patients experienced substantial relief of pain but only a small proportion achieved eradication of tumour (Table 3).

Dose Levels and Techniques. When patients were treated palliatively, simple techniques of treatment were used, frequently a parallel opposed pair of fields and radiation doses in the order of 30–35 gray in ten fractions over a period of 2 weeks. This regimen is associated with a low incidence of morbidity and can frequently carried out on an out-patient basis.

Radical Radiotherapy

For those patients suitable for radical radiotherapy the response rates achieved were much better. Patients were selected for radical x-ray treatment if they were found to

Table 4. Results of radical treatment (radiotherapy for inoperable tumours) of rectal cancer

Symptom	Complete response	Partial response	Failure
Pain	53.3%	33.3%	13.4%
Discharge	53.8%	30.8%	15.4%
Tumour	31.6%	52.6%	15.8%

Table 5. Results of radical treatment (radiotherapy for recurrent disease) of rectal cancer

Symptom	Complete response	Partial response	Failure
Pain	71.4%	19.1%	9.5%
Discharge	38.5%	46.1%	15.4%
Tumour	50.0%	37.5%	12.5%

have smaller tumours without any obvious evidence of metastatic disease. Correspondingly, such patients were frequently in better general condition. More complicated techniques of treatment were required for high-dose radiotherapy, frequently either a three-field beam-directed technique, each field being angled at 120° and a single anterior and two posterolateral fields being used. In other patients, a four-field box technique was employed. Dose levels in the order of 55 gray in 20 fractions in a period of 4 weeks are required for effective therapy of patients with inoperable or recurrent rectal carcinomas. It was of particular interest in patients with inoperable rectal tumours that with this form of treatment a local tumour control rate of over 30% could be achieved (Table 4). Similar response rates are seen in patients with recurrent tumour after previous definitive surgical operation. However, the assessment of complete tumour response is more difficult in these patients because of the previous surgery (Table 5).

Although these are patients with advanced disease and a correspondingly poor prognosis, long-term survival may be achieved for a few. In our experience patients with recurrent rectal cancer have a poorer prognosis than those with inoperable tumours, only 3.4% being alive at 5 years, compared with 15.8% of patients with inoperable disease.

Whilst a clinical trial comparing the results of treatment with combined chemotherapy and radiotherapy versus radiotherapy alone has not been conducted in Edinburgh, from serial analysis of patients treated by different methods with these high-dose techniques no advantage has been found from the combined technique in terms of either tumour response or overall survival. However, the morbidity of the combined regimen is substantially greater than that of radiotherapy alone. This supports the argument that, in large bowel cancer at least, 5-fluorouracil and radiotherapy act in an additive fashion rather than truly synergistically.

Other Radiotherapy Studies

Similar encouraging 5-year survival figures have been reported from other series in which patients with inoperable rectal carcinoma have been treated by radiotherapy. For example, Rao et al. (1978) have reported that 14% of a small group of 37 patients treated for inoperable and recurrent rectal carcinoma were alive at between 2 and 7 years after radiotherapy.

Thus it appears that in patients with symptom-producing disease, palliative radiotherapy can often be of great help in the alleviation of most distressing problems. Furthermore, in those patients suitable for high-dose radical radiotherapy worthwhile long-term survival may be achieved, particularly in patients with inoperable rectal cancer.

Patient Selection

One of the major problems in this group of patients is the selection of those suitable for high dose treatment. These high doses do give rise to definite morbidity, and it is essential therefore only to give radical treatment to patients with localized disease who may be potentially curable. However, conventional methods of detecting tumour spread are notoriously unreliable. For example, conventional radiology, biochemical tests of liver function and liver scans, together with ultrasonography, have a very high rate of false-negative results. CT scanning, should it be available, similarly has its limitations. It was with this in mind that a study was established in Edinburgh to assess the value of pretreatment serum CEA estimation as a means of selecting patients with inoperable and recurrent rectal cancers for either palliative or radical radiotherapy. The CEA was measured by a direct double-antibody radio immunoassay and the standard curve was shown to be parallel to that obtained with the British Standard for CEA, of which 0.004 U/ml are equivalent to 1 ng/ml in the Edinburgh assay. The upper limit of normal for the assay is 5 ng/ml or 0.02 British U/ml.

The outcome of treatment and the initial serum CEA level were correlated to see whether this investigation could be used to provide a more accurate guide to the most appropriate course of radiotherapy. As would have been anticipated, patients with high pretreatment levels of CEA had a relatively poor survival and inspection of the results showed that no patient with a pretreatment level greater than 75 ng/ml survived, despite radical treatment. A pretreatment CEA level of 75 ng/ml thus appeared to discriminate between those patients unlikely to benefit from radical radiotherapy and those more likely to respond well.

It must be emphasized that on conventional assessment, all these patients had been considered suitable for high dose treatment, and all had had liver scans or ultrasonography performed as a means of determining the presence of metastases. Interestingly, patients with very low CEA levels did not appear to fare as well as those with intermediate elevation, and it may be that this represents a group of patients who were non-secretors of CEA (Fig. 1).

The differences in survival between patients with moderately elevated CEA between 10 and 55 ng/ml and those with very high CEA levels was statistically significant at the 5% level.

Studies which have been conducted to investigate the sites of recurrence of rectal cancer in patients with advanced disease have suggested that when such patients are

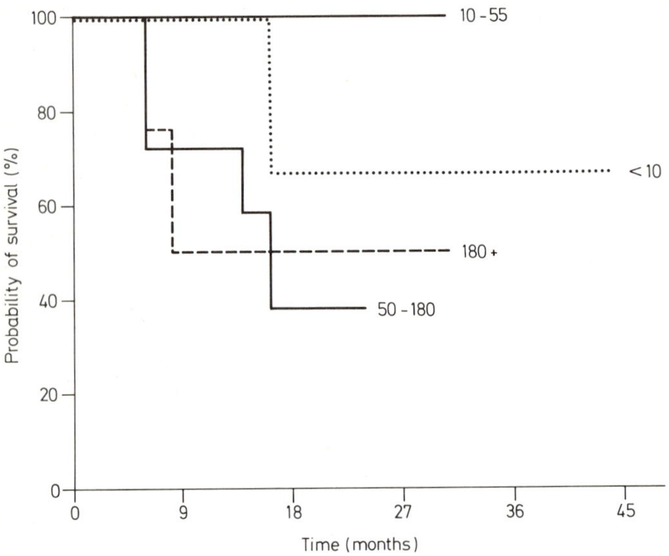

Fig. 1. Influence of CEA levels on survival after radical treatment of rectal cancer

treated a regional treatment technique should be adopted. For example, studies on patients with advanced rectal cancer who were subjected to planned second-look surgery have shown that in the majority of patients, local pelvic tumour recurrence remains the major problem (Gunderson and Sosin 1974). If therefore one is aiming to treat such disease primarily by radiotherapy, the whole of the area at risk must be included. However, if very large treatment fields are used there is a danger that the morbidity from treatment will increase due to the inclusion of large quantities of small bowel. Generally speaking, therefore, for carcinomas of the rectum fields are used which extend from the perineum to the sacral promontary.

High Dose Radiotherapy Studies

One of the major advantages of radiotherapy is that even in tumours very low in the rectum effective therapy will avoid the necessity for a colostomy, and the use of aggressive radiotherapy in such patients has been advocated strongly by Rider in Toronto (Rider 1975). He demonstrated in a group of patients who were initially included in a pre-operative radiotherapy trial, but who ultimately were treated only by radiotherapy because of subsequent refusal to have surgery, or assessment as unfit for operation, that the 5-year survival rate was twice as good as in a similar group of control patients treated by abdominoperineal excision alone. One of the difficulties in assessing results such as this is that this was not a truly randomized study and the method of case selection is not clear. Indeed, the opposite argument has been put forward by surgeons from the Toronto General Hospital, who analysed patients treated by abdominoperineal excision who were considered to be comparable with patients reported by Rider from the Princess Margaret Hospital, also in Toronto (Langer et al. 1977). It would be wrong to try to make too much of these individual claims, since none of the patients was prospectively randomized to receive one form of treatment or another. Nevertheless, it seems reasonable to suppose that radiotherapy may be as effective in curing a similar proportion of patients with low-lying tumours when abdominoperineal excision is necessary, particularly if adverse prognostic factors exist, such as tumour fixity. There is a considerable amount of evidence indicating that there is a marked difference in survival between patients with fixed tumours and those with mobile lesions. For example, a further study from the Princess Margaret Hospital, Toronto, which investigated the survival from the time of diagnosis of patients with tumours which were fixed and those which were considered fully mobile, demonstrated a significant difference between the two groups (Cummings 1978). Patients with mobile lesions had a 38% 5-year survival, whereas those with fixed tumours had a survival of only 19%. This work also shows that clinical assessment of the extent of tumour is of great prognostic value and may indicate that in the fixed group of tumours who are nevertheless deemed operable, other methods of treatment should be investigated.

Contact Radiotherapy and Interstitial Techniques

Another, quite different approach to low-lying tumours has been advised by Papillon (1975). This is the use of endocavitary irradiation. Papillon has suggested that radiotherapy given by a direct endocavitary technique may be the treatment of choice in selected patients. However, strict criteria must be observed. The tumour must be accessible, and must not be too large; indeed 5 cm is the maximum size that can be treated in this way. The tumour should be well differentiated and the degree of tumour infiltration must be small. Treatment is given by a 50 kV contact radiotherapy tube introduced into the rectum via a special sigmoidoscope.

The dose rate of this machine is high and treatment can be carried out within a few minutes in the out-patient clinic without an anaesthetic. Three to five applications are given and on each occasion a dose of between 25 and 40 gray is given. The total dose given is extremely high, of the order of 100–150 gray, and the total overall time is 5–6 weeks. This technique has yielded impressive results for Papillon. In 186 patients he claims a 5-year survival rate of 78%. The majority of his patients were deemed unsuitable for surgical resection, largely on account of medical illness. The results obtained in the treatment of polypoid tumours are particularly impressive, with a 91% local tumour control rate at times in excess of 18 months, and with only slightly poorer figures in patients with ulcerated tumours, although the number requiring subsequent surgery in this group is much higher. Obviously, this technique requires special equipment, which is costly, and of course it is only applicable to selected groups of patients.

An alternative approach is to carry out low rectal implantation. This is a technique which has been employed in Edinburgh during the past 2 years. Access to the lower rectum is obtained by means of an instrument such as the Park's anal retractor, which enables low-lying rectal tumours to be easily treated by local implantation. The advantage of this treatment is that apart from being effective, it is associated with a minimal degree of systemic upset and, particularly important in the elderly, with minimal bowel upset. Doses of the order of 60–70 gray in a period of 6–7 days are given. Obviously, the bowel requires careful preparation before the insertion of the needles. Careful patient selection is also necessary, since this treatment is really only suitable for the treatment of superficial tumours. However, it may be used on occasions to alleviate symptoms in patients who have developed further evidence of recurrent disease after previous treatment by radical external beam radiotherapy.

Developments in Radiotherapy

In recent years new methods of treating patients with rectal cancer by radiotherapy have been devised, the aim being to improve local tumour control rates whilst at the same time reducing treatment morbidity. These have included the use of innovative techniques, the use of hyperbaric oxygen as a radiosensitizer, and also fast neutron irradiation. One of the newer techniques of treatment which has been investigated has been the use of split-course radiotherapy. Most commonly, x-ray treatment is given on a regular daily basis over a period of 4–6 weeks. In split-course therapy the treatment is divided into two halves with a rest interval between. One of the principal advantages is that the gap in treatment allows improved recovery from acute radiation effects on normal tissues and may be associated with reduced radiation morbidity. In addition, during the rest interval continued tumour regression will occur. Claims have been made, following non-controlled investigations, that because of the reduced radiation morbidity associated with split-course treatment higher radiation doses may be given, leading to improved cure rates. Despite the use of these high doses, it was hoped that this treatment would be associated with reduced late radiation morbidity because of the repopulation taking place during the gap in treatment. Recent reports, however, have cast doubt on whether this is indeed the case. For example, a report from Canada suggested that in a small series of 24 patients, although the acute effects of treatment were minor, there was a 29% incidence of late major complications (Danjoux and Catton 1979). This study implied that the use of 5-fluorouracil, which was combined with the split-course treatment, might be responsible for the high incidence of late radiation morbidity. However, the same phenomena have been found in patients treated with x-ray treatment alone in Edinburgh. The regimen employed involved a dose of 35 gray in 3 weeks to large fields, including the whole pelvis, followed after a month's interval by a further dose of 35 gray given over a period of 2 weeks to reduced fields.

Only 19 patients have been treated with this regimen in Edinburgh, all of whom had inoperable tumours. The degree of local tumour control achieved was high, 52.6% of patients becoming free from any clinical evidence of tumour after therapy. Again, the immediate effects of radiotherapy were minimal. However, a very high proportion (21%) of patients developed major complications after therapy. This is very similar to the reported incidence of radiation morbidity in the Canadian study in which 5-fluorouracil was used as well as radiotherapy. What was found to be completely unacceptable in the Edinburgh series was the high death rate from radiation effects in patients in whom a complete tumour response had been achieved. No fewer than 15.8% of patients died as a result of serious radiation effects. Of the total of 19 patients only two are alive and free of disease or complications at present. Further reports have recently appeared indicating that similar problems are seen in the treatment of tumours at other sites (Parsans et al. 1980; Marcial et al. 1980), and it seems that there is little to support the use of split-course techniques in radiotherapy of large-bowel cancer. The benefit of reduced acute radiation morbidity is small and the incidence of late radiation complications is not reduced when similar local tumour control rates are obtained.

Table 6. Fast neutron trials in rectal cancer with the Edinburgh Cyclotron facility

Treatment	Number	Local control	Later recurrence
Photons	12	4	2
Neutrons	9	6	1

The potential of fast neutron therapy is currently under investigation in Edinburgh. One of the principal reasons for using this form of radiation in cancer treatment is that it is known from laboratory work that tissues which are not fully oxygenated are less sensitive to the lethal effects of x-rays, by a factor of about 3. Colonic and rectal tumours are known to contain numerous areas of necrosis and associated areas of hypoxia and it may be that such tumours contain as high a proportion as 15% of hypoxic yet viable cells. In addition, these tumours are known to have a great ability to repair sublethal damage inflicted by x-rays. It has been thought that these two factors may have contributed to some extent to the relative radioresistance of large-bowel cancer. The lethal effects of neutron irradiation are much less influenced by the absence of oxygen, and also it has been demonstrated that the ability of cells to repair sublethal radiation damage is markedly lower after neutron irradiation than after x-ray exposure. Thus, theoretically, neutrons appear to be able to overcome two of the principal reasons for radioresistance and therefore might prove more effective in the treatment of large bowel cancer.

To date, only small numbers of patients have been treated by neutrons in Edinburgh, but pilot studies demonstrated that the relief of symptoms appears to be at least as good as that achieved by conventional radiotherapy (Table 6).

Following a period of pilot work in which dose-ranging studies were conducted to find a satisfactory dose level with neutrons, which would be effective yet associated with a low level of morbidity, randomized clinical studies have been undertaken. As yet, the number of patients included in the studies is very small but it appears so far that there is very little difference between the modalities of treatment in the achievement of local tumour control. However, it is certainly far too early to draw any conclusions about the possible role of neutron irradiation in the management of this disease.

Encouraging reports have also been reported following the use of hyperbaric oxygen with x-ray therapy (Dische and Senanayake 1972). Further studies are being conducted with drugs which act as hypoxic cell sensitizers, such as metronidozole and misonidazole.

Combined Surgery and Radiotherapy

One of the most exciting developments currently being investigated is a combined approach in which surgery and radiotherapy are being employed together in an attempt to improve cure rates in patients with operable disease.

Radiotherapy may be employed either before or after a surgical procedure, and either low dose or high dose treatment may be given. The problem with postoperative therapy is that any treatment given will not deal with cells which may potentially disseminate at operation. It will, however, have some effect on local tumour recurrence. Only high dose radiotherapy may be effective in these circumstances. The

advantage of giving postoperative therapy is that exploration of the patient has been carried out and definitive information is available concerning the extent of tumour, enabling accurate postoperative treatment to be given. However, following surgery great care must be taken in the technique of treatment used and the dosage employed, as otherwise there will be considerable postoperative radiation morbidity.
There is a great deal of interest at present in the potential of pre-operative radiotherapy, which may take either the form of high dose treatment or low dose irradiation. High dose radiotherapy will certainly influence the tumour and may make operation easier. However, following such treatment it is necessary for there to be a delay before an operation can be performed to allow recovery from the immediate radiation reaction. This delay might allow re-growth of tumour to occur and perhaps metastases to develop before surgery is performed.

Low Dose Pre-operative Radiotherapy

One of the advantages of low dose treatment is that immediate operation is possible after such therapy, and it does not exclude further treatment after surgery should this be necessary. In addition, all the evidence suggests that there is no increased morbidity or mortality associated with this form of therapy. One of the first reports suggesting possible benefit from low-dose treatment came from the Memorial Hospital in 1959 (Stearns et al. 1959). This was a report of a retrospective study of patients treated for rectal carcinoma between 1939 and 1951. The patients in this study were not randomized and often the reasons for giving the treatment were not clear. However, it was found that patients with Dukes' C lesions of the bowel had a better 5-year survival if they had received a course of low dose pre-operative radiotherapy, and that this improved survival was maintained at 10 years. A subsequent prospective study carried out at the same centre with a similar treatment regimen has failed, however, to confirm these results (Stearns et al. 1974). Nevertheless, stimulated by this work, in 1964 the Veterans Administration Surgical Group in the United States of America began a prospective controlled randomized trial of the use of low dose pre-operative radiotherapy in clinically operable patients with carcinoma of the rectum. Only male patients were investigated, and when the study was closed in 1969 a total of 700 patients had been included (Roswit et al. 1975). One of the striking features found in this trial was a reduction in the incidence of lymph nodes involved by tumour in patients who had undergone pre-operative radiotherapy and, in addition, survival rates were found to be better in the irradiated group, especially in those who required an abdominoperineal excision. At one time it was suggested that this difference in survival was statistically significant. However, the organizers of the study at present urge that caution should be exercised in interpreting these results. It is felt that when particular subgroups of patients within the trial are compared, any differences demonstrated should be expected to show higher levels of statistical significance than the conventional values before they are considered real (Higgins 1979). Nevertheless, these figures are highly suggestive. In a group of 180 patients examined at autopsy, there was indeed a statistically significant difference in the presence of cancer at the time of death in patients managed by pre-operative radiotherapy compared with those managed by surgery alone. This interesting study stimulated the establishment of an investigation of pre-operative radiotherapy in the United Kingdom, under the auspices of the Medical Research Council. It was agreed that the regime according to which 20 gray is given in ten treatments, followed by surgery as soon thereafter as possible, as practised in the Veterans Administration study, should be repeated and compared with a single dose of 5 gray. On theoretical grounds this should be effective in dealing with those tumour cells most likely to be disseminated at surgery, and is attractive in that it reduces the delay in carrying out definitive surgical resection to a minimum. Following the commencement of the MRC trial, a study had been reported from Toronto which has indicated that patients with Dukes' C tumours receiving a single dose of 5 gray pre-operative radiotherapy fared significantly better than those treated by surgery only (Rider et al. 1977). However, the number of patients in this trial is small, raising some doubt as to the statistical validity of the result.

When the MRC rectal cancer study was closed, 824 patients had been included and were available for analysis. The patients had been contributed from 17 centres throughout the United Kingdom. Preliminary analysis has shown that in this trial also the incidence of involved nodes has been reduced from 44.6% in the controlled group to 35.9% in patients undergoing the multiple-dose pre-operative course of treatment. This difference, however, does not quite achieve conventional levels of statistical significance. What is interesting in this study, however, is that the incidence of uninvolved nodes has also been reduced in those undergoing multiple-dose treatment and that this reduction is statistically significant. A further interesting feature is that in patients undergoing multiple-dose treatment there was a statistically significantly greater proportion of small tumours under 4 cm in size. This preliminary evidence indicates that these low doses of radiotherapy do have a biological effect on the tumour. As yet, there is no evidence from the MRC trial that this treatment is in any way associated with increased morbidity or mortality after surgery.

Although low dose radiotherapy does produced measurable biological effects on rectal cancer, there is still some doubt concerning whether this form of pre-operative radiotherapy makes a real contribution to improved survival rates. This in turn has stimulated a re-appraisal of the potential value of high-dose pre-operative radiotherapy.

High Dose Pre-Operative Radiotherapy

There is substantial evidence that high dose radiotherapy influences rectal cancer and, even in patients with inoperable disease, may be associated with long-term survival (Rider 1975). However, it might be that the use of pre-operative radiotherapy, perhaps with high dose treatment, should be given only to those patients known to have an increased risk of local recurrence and metastasis, for example, patients with fixed tumours or those which are locally advanced yet still deemed operable. There can be no doubt that these patients do fare much worse following surgery than those with earlier, mobile tumours. This was demonstrated clearly in the University of Minnesota study of planned re-operation for patients with locally advanced tumours (Gunderson and Sosin 1974).

No fewer than 70% of patients examined in this way developed subsequent evidence of recurrent tumour. In nearly half these recurrence was only in the form of local pelvic tumour. It seems reasonable, therefore, to suppose that giving radiotherapy in these circumstances might substantially reduce the problem of local recurrence and contribute to increased survival rates. As yet, no randomized clinical trial of any size has been conducted to test this hypothesis. A non-randomized investigation recently reported from America has shown, in patients deemed to have a curative resection performed after high dose radiotherapy, that the incidence of local recurrence was nil at 5 years, and the 5-year survival rate was 53% (Stevens et al. 1976). The authors state that this compares with a historic 5-year survival rate of 38% in the same hospital. In addition, patients with inoperable tumours, in whom it was planned to carry out a resection later should the disease become operable, were examined. The 5-year survival rate for this group was 12.5%, which is no better than the results of treating inoperable patients by radical radiotherapy alone in the Edinburgh series. Thus, in patients with truly inoperable tumours very careful assessment is necessary before surgery is considered, particularly as this may necessitate the formation of a colostomy. It would perhaps, therefore, be better to reserve resection for patients in whom there is a good but incomplete response to radiotherapy. It may be that patients who do well following radical radiotherapy for inoperable tumours may not need surgery at all.

Postoperative Radiotherapy

Postoperative radiotherapy is the least attractive of the combined radiotherapy/surgery options. Although this treatment should be capable of reducing local tumour recurrence in selected patients, it may be associated with severe radiation morbidity and even mortality. This was clearly shown in a non-randomized study conducted at the MD Anderson Hospital in Houston (Withers and Romsdahl 1977), in which the local recurrence rate was reduced to only 4.4% following postoperative radiotherapy, compared with 21% in those patients treated by surgery only. However, the incidence of radiation morbidity was considerable. It is almost certainly better to give postoperative radiotherapy immediately after surgery when the residual disease is minimal than to wait for the development of gross tumour recurrence; our experience in Edinburgh shows that even radical radiotherapy in these circumstances is much less effective.

Conclusions

There can be no doubt that radiotherapy has a role to play in the management of patients with carcinoma of the rectum. It is certainly of great palliative benefit in those patients with disease which is either recurrent after previous surgery or deemed inoperable. In addition, in this group of patients worthwile 5-year survival rates may be achieved in selected patients given radical radiotherapy. However, careful selection must be adopted in choosing patients for radical treatment. In other highly selected patients local methods of radiotherapy, either by endocavitary irradiation or by local implantation techniques, may also prove to be of great value. These certainly have the advantage of a low rate of morbidity with a high level of tumour control.

There is no evidence at present that radiotherapy is superior to surgery in the treatment of operable tumours. Currently the field of greatest interest is the use of combined techniques of management in which radiotherapy is given in conjunction with surgery. Most of the evidence suggests that pre-operative radiotherapy is preferable to postoperative radiotherapy. As yet, the optimum dose of pre-operative radiation is not clear. The results which are available do suggest that low-dose pre-operative radiotherapy does have a definite biological effect on rectal cancer, and it may well be shown in the future that this form of adjuvant treatment will lead to improved cure rates in patients with operable disease.

References

Arnott SJ (1975) The value of combined 5-fluorouracil and X-ray therapy in the palliation of locally recurrent and inoperable rectal carcinoma. Clin Radiol 26: 177–181

Cummings BJ (1978) Radiation therapy in rectal cancer. Can J Surg 21: 44–46

Danjoux CE, Catton GE (1979) Delayed complications in colo-rectal carcinoma treated by combination radiotherapy and 5-fluorouracil – Eastern cooperative oncology group (ECOG) pilot study. Int J Radiat Oncol Biol Phys 5: 311–315

Dische S, Senanayake F (1972) Radiotherapy using hyperbaric oxygen in the palliation of carcinoma of colon and rectum. Clin Radiol 23: 512–518

Gunderson LL, Sosin H (1974) Areas of failure found at reoperation (second or symptomatic look) following "curative surgery" for adenocarcinoma of the rectum. Cancer 34: 1278–1292

Heidelberger C, Griesbach L, Montag BJ, Mooren D, Cruz O, Schnitzer RJ, Gruneberg E (1958) Studies on fluorinated pyrimidines. II. Effects on transplanted tumours. Cancer Res 18: 305–317

Higgins GA (1979) Adjuvant radiation therapy in colon cancer. International Advances in Surgical Oncology 2: 1–24

Langer B, Toree EB, Patel S (1977) Radical radiotherapy versus abdominoperineal resection as primary treatment of carcinoma of the lower rectum. Can Med Assoc J 117: 1183–1184

Marcial VA, Hanley JA, Chang G, Davis LW and Moscol JA (1980) Split-course radiation therapy of carcinoma of the nasopharynx: results of a national collaborative clinical trial of the radiation therapy oncology group. Int J Radiat Oncol Biol Phys 6: 409–414

Moertel CG, Childs DS Jr, Reitemeier RJ, Colby MY, Holbrook M (1969) 5-fluorouracil and radiotherapy for gastrointestinal cancer. Lancet 2: 865–867

Papillon J (1975) Intracavitary irradiation of early rectal cancer for cure – a series of 186 cases. Cancer 36: 696–701

Parsons JT, Thar TL, Bova FJ, Million RR (1980) An evaluation of split-course irradiation for pelvic malignancies. Int J Radiat Oncol Biol Phys 6: 175–181

Rider WD (1975) Is the Miles operation really necessary for the treatment of rectal cancer? The Gordon Richards Memorial Lecturer. J Can Assoc Radiol 26: 167–175

Rider WD, Palmer JA, Mahoney LJ, Robertson CT (1977) Pre-operative irradiation in operable cancer of the rectum: report of the Toronto trial. Can J Surg 20: 335–338

Rao AR, Kagan AR, Chan PYM, Gilbert HA, Nussbaum H (1978) Effectiveness of local radiotherapy in colorectal carcinoma. Cancer 42: 1082–1086

Roswit B, Higgins GA Jr, Keehn RJ (1975) Pre-operative irradiation for carcinoma of the rectum and recto-sigmoid colon – report of the National Veterans Administration randomised study. Cancer 35: 1597–1602

Stearns MW Jr, Deddish MR, Quan SH (1959) Preoperative roentgen therapy for cancer of the rectum. Surg Gynaecol Obstet 109: 225–229

Stearns MW Jr, Deddish MR, Quan SH (1974) Preoperative roentgen therapy for cancer of the rectum and recto-sigmoid. Surg Gynaecol Obstet 138: 584–586

Stevens KR, Allan CV, Fletcher WS (1976) Preoperative radiotherapy for adenocarcinoma of the recto-sigmoid. Cancer 37: 2866–2869

Vietti T, Eggerding F, Valeriote F (1971) Combined effect of X-radiation and 5-fluorouracil on survival of transplanted leukaemia cells. J Natl Cancer Inst 47: 865–870

Williams IG, Horwitz H (1956) The primary treatment of adenocarcinoma of the rectum by high voltage roentgen rays (1000 kV). Am J Roentgenol 76: 919–923

Withers HR, Romsdahl MM (1977) Post-operative radiotherapy for adenocarcinoma of the rectum and recto-sigmoid. Int J Radiat Oncol Biol Phys 2: 1069–1074

Chemotherapy

J. M. A. Whitehouse

CRC Medical Oncology Unit, Southampton General Hospital,
Southampton S09 4XY, United Kingdom

Carcinomas of the colon and rectum have certain characteristics which indicate a potential role for chemotherapy in their management. Principal among these is the fact that the disease appears widespread in a majority of cases. This can be concluded from the failure of local forms of management – primarily surgery alone – to cure more than 30% of cases overall, despite an apparently curative resection. Once bowel is resected, the Dukes' staging system can be used as a crude indicator of the risk of subsequent clinical relapse, but for the patient with demonstrable metastases at the time of operation, the median survival is less than 1 year. This compares with a 5-year survival rate of 30% for patients with apparently localized Dukes' C tumours.

Since colorectal carcinomas are common, any response to treatment should be readily evaluable. In addition, 70% of lesions are found within a region extending down from the sigmoid colon to the lower rectum, so that clinical or endoscopic evaluation of tumour masses is relatively easy. Unfortunately, this does not facilitate assessment of the effects of chemotherapy, for the primary tumour is often resected, and while intra-abdominal disease may be clearly defined at the initial operation subsequent assessment is dependent on the findings of non-invasive, and often much less sensitive, techniques.

Newer techniques of abdominal ultrasound, laparoscopy, and CT scanning may be helpful in contributing to a broad assessment of response, but it can be appreciated that the precision of documentation of that assessment may vary considerably between institutions, and indeed between clinicians. Survival is the simplest common denominator by which to judge response to therapy. However, it is now appreciated that comparative studies must be stratified, at least for such factors as site of lesion, Dukes' stage, sex of patient, and operative procedure. If this is not done, the risk of comparing non-balanced heterogeneous groups is increased, and with it the hazard of drawing unjustified conclusions. This is particularly so when trials containing relatively small numbers of patients are reported.

Many collections of data relating to chemotherapy administration in patients with colorectal carcinoma suffer from the consequences of neglecting these factors in trial design and analysis. However, within the last years a number of carefully conducted studies have been reported, so that it is possible to derive a realistic appraisal of the influence of available anticancer agents on the natural history of tumours arising in the colon and rectum. Unfortunately, the one factor which would lend great encouragement to the role of chemotherapy, namely a drug producing a high response rate, has not so far emerged. Among those patients whose tumours do respond an improvement in survival cannot be unequivocally attributed to chemotherapy.

Recent Results in Cancer Research, Vol. 83

Some 40 single agents have been evaluated with varying degrees of thoroughness, and always in patients with advanced disease.

Single Agents

The very real problems of assessing a reduction of tumour size in colorectal carcinoma has meant that meaningful single-agent response data for a range of commonly used drugs are available only in part. 5-Fluorouracil (5-FU) has almost by default become the standard against which any new drug should be measured. In its favour is the fact that at conventional doses toxicity is predominantly that of temporary nausea and bone marrow suppression. Furthermore, where used alone 5-FU can produce an objective response at 2 months of between 17% and 20%, and a median response duration of 5 months (Moertel 1975). Although oral preparations are available, at least two clinical studies have shown intravenous administration of 5-FU to produce superior results (Hahn et al. 1975; Bateman et al. 1975). Even so, out-patient management is simple and this undoubtedly favours its selection for therapy over drugs with equal activity or greater toxicity. The activities of some agents, including some recently assessed are compared in Table 1.

Of the antimetabolites, methotrexate has been reported to have produced a 15% response rate in a selected series of 128 patients (Livingston and Carter 1970) but only a 5% response rate in a smaller series with stricter response criteria (Moertel 1975).

One of the newer antimetabolites, Baker's antifol (Triazinate), has antifolate activity. Its predominant toxicities are myelosuppression, dermatitis, and mucositis. In a phase I study at the MD Anderson Hospital in which doses of 10–250 mg/m^2 were given daily for 5 days, some antitumour activity was shown in colorectal carcinomas. Life-threatening toxicity was seen in patients with impaired liver function (Rodriguez et al. 1976). Rodriguez et al. (1977), using a dose of 250 mg/m^2 daily for 3 days later attained 4 partial remissions in 25 patients with colorectal carcinoma. The South-Western Oncology Group, in a phase II study of 30 patients who had failed to improve with previous therapy, recorded 3 partial responses (Padilla et al. 1978) in 29 evaluable patients who had previously been treated with 5-FU either alone or in combination with mitomycin C or methyl-CCNU.

Table 1. Response to single agents in advanced colorectal carcinoma

Reference	Agent	Response (%)
Carter 1976	5-FU	15–21
Livingston and Carter 1970	Methotrexate	15
Moertel 1975	Methotrexate	5
Rodriguez et al. 1977	Baker's Antifolate	16
Buroker et al. 1979	Ftorafur	11
DiBenedetto et al. 1978	Melphalan	0
Nair et al. 1980	Fluorodopan	6
Douglass et al. 1978	Methyl-CCNU	15
Moertel 1976	Mitomycin C	16
Carter and Friedman 1974	Adriamycin	9

A fluorinated pyrimidine analogue of 5-FU, ftorafur, was reported to have significant activity in large-bowel cancer (Blokhina et al. 1972). The lack of myelosuppression associated with its use in phase I trials is comparable to the bone marrow sparing of 5-FU infusions. Since the active metabolite of ftorafur is 5-FU the decrease in myelosuppression is attributed to a slow release of 5-FU from the biological system. No responses have been seen in patients who previously received treatment with 5-FU (Buroker et al. 1977). In 84 previously untreated patients receiving ftorafur at a dosage of 2.25 g/m^2 per day for 5 days and repeated at 3-weekly intervals, regressions were noted in 9/84 patients. The median survival of responders was 32 weeks, but responders only survived 5 weeks longer than non-responders. The major dose-limiting toxicity was that involving the central nervous system (Buroker et al. 1979). Since the active metabolite of ftorafur is 5-FU it is inevitable that response rates will be either similar to or inferior to those obtained with 5-FU.

None of the alkylating agents appears to have greater activity than 5-FU. DiBenedetto et al. (1978), in a phase II study, treated 25 patients, all of whom had failed to improve with previous alternative chemotherapy, with melphalan 0.25 mg/kg orally for 4 days every 28 days. No responses were seen. However, 24 of the 25 patients had been previously treated with methyl-CCNU and all had received 5-FU.

Fluorodopan [5-(2′-fluoroethyl-2′-chloroethyl)-amino-6-methyluracil] is a derivative of uracil mustard. This was given to 17 previously treated patients with advanced carcinoma of the colon or rectum, but a partial remission was seen in only 1 patient (Nair et al. 1980).

The related drugs, the nitrosoureas, produce similarly disappointing response rates of 10%–15% (Moertel 1976). Recently methyl-CCNU was compared in a large study (Douglass et al. 1978) with 5-FU. The response rates were identical, but 24% of the patients treated with methyl-CCNU had severe or life-threatening haematological toxicity. Nausea and vomiting were also more severe among this group.

Other drugs, such as rubidazone (Fraile et al. 1978) pyrazofurin (Carroll et al. 1979) ICRF 159 (Marciniak et al. 1975) metronidazole (Frytak et al. 1978), maytansine (O'Connell et al. 1978) and 2-2′-anhydro-1-beta-arabino-furanosyl 5-fluorocytosine (Kemeny et al. 1978), have all been shown to produce little response. Only mitomycin C approaches the activity of 5-FU (Crooke and Bradnes 1976), but its toxicity does not make it an attractive alternative; and the potent antitumour antibiotic adriamycin has an even lower response rate, of about 9% (Carter and Friedman 1974).

Despite the very intensive study of single agents in this common condition over a period of many years, 5-FU remains the best documented, and the most consistent in producing the highest response rates. Recent correspondence (Ansfield and Greenspan 1979) proposes the importance of the relationship between 5-FU dosage at levels producing appreciable toxicity and maximum therapeutic effect. Whatever the theory, the reality is that survival is only marginally improved when disease regression is produced by one of the available drugs at present.

Combination Chemotherapy

The poor overall response rates documented for single agents do not augur well for their use in combination. None of the more active agents has recognized synergistic properties with other compounds, and although many different combinations have

Table 2. Response to combined chemotherapy in advanced colorectal carcinoma

Refernce	Agents	No. of patients	Response (%)
Moertel et al. 1975	5-FU, MeCCNU, VCR	39	43.5
Moertel 1978	5-FU, MeCCNU, VCR	137	27
Joss et al. 1979	5-FU, MeCCNU, VCR	52	11
Taylor et al. 1979	CTX, UCR, MTX	20	20
Buroker et al. 1977, 1979	5-FU, Mito C	136	18
	5-FU, MeCCNU	133	16
Krause et al. 1979	5-FU, Mito C	51	33
Douglass et al. 1978	5-FU, CTX	87	5
	5-FU, 6-TG	77	12
Gough et al. 1979	5-FU, melphalan	9	22
Haller et al. 1978	5-FU, ADR, Mito C	35	17
Hall et al. 1978	Baker's antifol, ADR	10	20
Buroker et al. 1977, 1979	Ftorafur, Mito C	26	27
	Ftorafur, MeCCNU	26	15
Belt and Stephens 1979	Ftorafur, MeCCNU	36	15

5-FU, 5-fluorouracil; ADR, adriamycin; Mito C, mitomycin C; CTX, cyclophosphamide; MeCCNU, methyl-CCNU; 6-TG, 6-thioguanine

been studied, as might be expected, few show remarkable improvements in response rates compared with 5-FU used alone. Some of the more recently studied combinations are listed in Table 2. In 1975 Moertel et al. reported a 43.5% response rate for 5-FU, vincristine, and methyl-CCNU, as against 19% for 5-FU alone, and this has become the standard against which other combinations are assessed. Disappointingly, despite the improved response rate recorded for the multi-drug arm, no survival improvement could be shown over that for 5-FU alone. Response rates approaching these figures have been recorded by other groups (Baker et al. 1976; Falkson and Falkson 1976; Kisner et al. 1979).

However, this same group from the Mayo Clinic (Moertel 1978), analysing an expanded population of 137 patients, showed their response rates to have fallen from 43.5% to 27%. Several uncontrolled studies of vincristine, methyl-CCNU and 5-FU, and of 5-FU and methyl-CCNU have now been reported (Table 2). Only in Moertel's own studies did the addition of vincristine show a particular advantage. The response rate was 27% for the three-drug regimen, and only 16% among 61 patients treated with 5-FU and methyl-CCNU. In a total of 489 patients from six studies treated with 5-FU and methyl-CCNU, 19% overall achieved complete remission, while 25% of 358 patients in five collected studies treated with 5-FU, methyl-CCNU and vincristine did so – a difference too small to be of real therapeutic significance.

In a preliminary report of nine evaluable patients treated with melphalan combined with 5-FU, two showed objective responses (Gough et al. 1979). In another study 5-FU was combined with mitomycin C, and 9 patients out of 51 (33%) showed tumour regression (Krause et al. 1979). The median duration of response was 5 months, but seven patients survived for 1 year or more. However, three patients developed severe respiratory insufficiency and the suggestion was made by these authors that this combination might cause pulmonary toxicity. This complication was not reported by the South-West Oncology Group (Crooke and Bradnes 1976), who compared 5-FU infusions in combination with either mitomycin C or methyl-CCNU. The response rates of these combinations were 18% and 16%, respectively, but in this case the median survival for all treated patients was 43 weeks on both arms, illustrating the difficulty of comparing results from different centres.

The Eastern Cooperative Oncology Group randomized 316 patients to receive 5-FU given orally or intravenously, 5-FU given orally in combination with cyclophosphamide or 6-thioguanine, or the drug methyl-CCNU alone (Douglass et al. 1978). Response rates among patients who had received no prior chemotherapy were 18% to oral 5-FU, 15% to intravenous 5-FU or methyl-CCNU, 12% to 5-FU and 6-thioguanine, and 5% to 5-FU and cyclophosphamide. A 3% response rate only was seen in previously treated or relapsed patients receiving cross-over therapy.

When used as a single agent for colorectal carcinoma adriamycin has only low activity. However, the combination of 5-FU, adriamycin, and mitomycin C (FAM) has been widely studied in the treatment of gastric cancer, and has produced response rates as high as 50%. When the FAM regimen (5-FU, adriamycin, and mitomycin C) was given to 35 patients with advanced measurable colorectal carcinoma, 6 (17%) patients had objective regression in tumour size (Haller et al. 1978). Baker's antifolate was combined with adriamycin in the treatment of ten patients (Hall et al. 1978). Two patients with pulmonary metastases achieved partial remission. Pharmacokinetic studies carried out by this group revealed that Baker's antifolate levels were prolonged, apparently due to an adriamycin effect on the plasma elimination of that drug.

Since combinations of methyl-CCNU and 5-FU have produced some of the better responses recorded, and since ftorafur has less of a myelosuppressive effect than 5-FU, the combination of ftorafur and methyl-CCNU is of interest. However, when this combination was used in the treatment of 36 patients (Belt and Stephens 1979) there was significant toxicity and only 14.7% of patients achieved a partial response.

None of these studies shows any significant improvement over the response rates achieved with 5-FU alone. In 1978, Moertel wrote:

. . . it must be concluded that there is no chemotherapy approach to gastrointestinal carcinoma valuable enough to justify application of standard clinical treatment.

And in subsequent correspondence (Moertel 1979): I cannot accept the contention that gastrointestinal patients' most ideal and frequently only opportunity to receive beneficial chemotherapy should be wasted by exposure to routine 5-FU at either toxic or non-toxic doses. On the other hand I do think that pessimism about treatment for these patients can be dispelled by thoughtfully designed clinical research programmes which offer the hope of realistic gain.

It is to be hoped that the established value of the well-structured clinical trial in improving disease management will encourage this approach. The empirically treated patient remains a subjective impression in whom there is no prospect of evaluating either benefit or harm.

Intra-Arterial Therapy

The liver is a common site for metastases in patients with colorectal carcinoma. Indeed, more than 50% of all patients may have liver involvement. The response to intravenous therapy is poor, and the pain and jaundice resulting from hepatic infiltration respond poorly to palliative measures. Drugs such as 5-FU, and

5-fluorodeoxyuridine (5-FUDR) are both metabolized in the liver, so that delivery of either of these drugs via the hepatic artery might be anticipated to ensure high tumour levels. The most comprehensive study is that reported by Ansfield et al. (1975), in which 419 patients received percutaneous arterial infusion chemotherapy for liver metastases. An initial 3-week course of intra-arterial 5-FU administered through a transbrachial catheter was followed by weekly intravenous 5-FU. Responses were seen in 55% of patients, with a median survival of 7.3 months. Toxicity was predictably less than might be anticipated following administration by continuous intravenous infusion, and consisted of gastrointestinal side-effects in about 10% of patients and myelosuppression in less than 5%. The Central Oncology Group (Grage et al. 1977) randomized 61 patients to receive either arterial perfusion or intravenous 5-FU. Patients were stratified prior to randomization and subsequently received weekly 5-FU as maintenance therapy until progression. No advantage could be demonstrated for the intra-arterial therapy. Although the response rate was 34%, compared with 23% for those treated with intravenous therapy alone, the median survival in the latter group was 13.3 months, as against 10 months among those receiving intra-arterial therapy. A portable infusion pump linked to a catheter placed in the hepatic artery following insertion via the brachial artery permitted prolonged and continuous percutaneous arterial infusion therapy (Oberfield et al. 1979). Between 1969 and 1976 a total of 60 patients were treated with a 10-day course of 5-FU and then discharged home, receiving 5-FUDR by continuous arterial infusion through a chronometric infusion pump. Complete responses were seen in 15% of patients and partial responses in 39%, but the median survival from the onset of treatment was still low, 8.5 and 6.9 months, respectively. Patients treated previously with 5-FU intravenously did, however, respond to intra-arterial chemotherapy, 13% achieving a complete response and 54% partial response.

Following tumour resection hepatic metastases may represent the only site of detectable residual disease. Patt et al. (1981) used hepatic arterial infusion of 5-FUDR and mitomycin C in the treatment of 55 such patients. Three complete responses and 21 partial responses were recorded. Hepatic arterial occlusions occurred inadvertently in 13 patients and deliberately in 11. The median survival for all patients was 11 months; however, the median survival for patients with arterial occlusion was 15 months, compared with 8 months for those without arterial occlusion.

The problems of this technique are essentially those relating to systemic toxicity and to the catheter itself. These include breakage at some point in the catheter and infection at the site of insertion. Complete or partial thrombosis of the artery may also occur.

These various findings are encouraging in terms of response, and improvements in technology make continuous arterial infusion with portable pumps a practical proposition for the ambulant patient. As yet, despite significant responses in hepatic metastases there has not yet been a significant improvement in survival.

Adjuvant Chemotherapy for Large Bowel Cancer

Great interest has been aroused in the potential for adjuvant chemotherapy in colorectal carcinoma. Carter (1979), in his review of the role of 5-FU as adjuvant chemotherapy for large bowel cancer, has examined the studies reported by Higgins (1976) and Higgins et al. (1971, 1978), Dwight et al. (1973), Lawrence et al. (1978)

Grage et al. (1977), and Grossi et al. (1977). In 2287 patients distributed throughout these randomized studies no advantage could be demonstrated for 5-FU adjuvant therapy over control treatment with no chemotherapy. He concludes that no properly designed prospectively randomized trial of 5-FU adjuvant treatment has shown statistically significant benefit.

However, since that review Taylor et al. (1979) have reported the results of hepatic perfusion of 5-FU via the umbilical vein. This is a randomized study of 154 consecutive patients. Eleven were excluded because of either technical problems with the infusion or the demonstration of metastases at the time of operation. Seventy-three patients underwent surgical resection alone and 66 received liver perfusion. Long-term analysis is not yet possible. However, at the time of reporting 23 patients had died in the control group, compared with seven in the perfusion group. Thirteen of the control patients had developed liver metastases, compared with two in the perfusion group. It is premature to judge these results too optimistically, but this technique obviously merits further study. By comparison, the routine administration of intravenous 5-FU as adjuvant treatment for patients undergoing resection of apparently localized colorectal tumours cannot be justified at present.

References

Ansfield FJ, Greenspan EM (1979) 5-Fluorouracil for gastrointestinal cancer. N Engl J Med 301:328

Ansfield FJ, Ramirez G, Davis HL, Wirtanen GW, Johnson RO, Bryan GT, Manalo FB, Borden EC, Davis TE, Esmaili ME (1975) Further clinical studies with intrahepatic arterial infusion with 5-fluorouracil. Cancer 36:2413–2417

Baker LH, Talley RW, Matter R, Lahane DE, Ruffner BW, Jones SE, Morrison FS, Stephens RL, Gehan EA, Vaitkevicius VK (1976) Phase III comparison of the treatment of advanced gastrointestinal cancer with bolus weekly 5-FU vs methyl-CCNU plus bolus weekly 5-FU. Cancer 38:1

Bateman J, Irwin L, Pugh R, Cassidy F, Weiner J (1975) Comparison of intravenous and oral administration of 5-fluorouracil for colorectal carcinoma. Proc Am Soc Clin Oncol 16:242

Belt RJ, Stephens R (1979) Phase I–II study of ftorafur and methyl-CCNU in advanced colorectal cancer. Cancer 44:869–872

Blokhina NG, Vozny EK, Garin AM (1972) Results of treatment of malignant tumors with ftorafur. Cancer 30:390–392

Buroker T, Miller A, Baker L, McKenzie M, Samson M, Vaitkevicius VK (1977) Phase II clinical trial of ftorafur in 5-fluorouracil-refractory colorectal cancer. Cancer Treat Rep 61:1579

Buroker T, Padilla F, Groppe C, Guy G, Quagliana J, McCracken J, Vaitkevicius VK, Hoogstraten B, Heilbrun L (1979) Phase II evaluation of ftorafur in previously untreated colorectal cancer. Cancer 44:48–51

Carroll DS, Kemeny NE, Gralla RJ (1979) Phase II evaluation of pyrazofurin in patients with advanced colorectal carcinoma. Cancer Treat Rep 63:139–140

Carter SK (1976) Large bowel cancer – The current status of treatment. J Natl Cancer Inst 56:3

Carter SK (1979) 5-Fluorouracil as adjuvant chemotherapy for large bowel cancer: Is it appropriate for routine community use? Cancer Chemother Pharmacol 2:81–84

Carter SK, Friedman M (1974) Integration of chemotherapy into combined-modality treatment of solid tumors. II. Large bowel carcinoma. Cancer Treat Rev 1:111–129

Crooke S, Bradnes W (1976) Mitomycin-C: A review. Cancer Treat Rev 3:121–139

DiBenedetto J, Moayeri H, Evans JT, Mittelman A (1978) Phase II study of melphalan in colorectal carcinoma. Cancer Treat Rep 62: 1401–1402
Douglass HO, Lavin PT, Woll J, Conroy JF, Carbone P (1978) Chemotherapy of advanced measurable colon and rectal carcinoma with oral 5-fluorouracil, alone or in combination with cyclophosphamide or 6-thioguanine, with intravenous 5-fluorouracil or beta-2′-deoxythioguanosine or with oral 3(4-methyl-cyclohexyl)-1(2-chlorethyl)-1-nitrosourea. Cancer 42: 2538–2545
Dwight RW, Humphrey EW, Higgins GA et al. (1973) FUDR as an adjuvant to surgery in cancer of the large bowel. J Surg Oncol 5: 243
Falkson G, Falkson HC (1976) Fluorouracil, methyl-CCNU and vincristine in cancer of the colon. Cancer 38: 1468
Fraile RJ, Samson MK, Buroker TR, O'Bryan R, Baker LH, Vaitkevicius VT (1978) Clinical trial of rubidazone in advanced squamous cell carcinoma of the lung and adenocarcinoma of the large intestine. Cancer Treat Rep 62: 1599
Frytak S, Moertel CG, Childs DS, Schutt AJ, Albers JW (1978) Phase II study of metronidazole therapy for advanced colorectal carcinoma. Cancer Treat Rep 62: 483–485
Gough IR, Furnival CM, Burnett W (1979) Melphalan and 5-fluorouracil in advanced gastrointestinal carcinoma: A preliminary report. Cancer Treat Rev 6: 127–129
Grage TD, Metter GE, Cornell JN et al. (1977) Adjuvant chemotherapy with 5-fluorouracil after surgical resection of colorectal carcinoma (COG protocol 7041): A preliminary report. Am J Surg 133: 59–66
Grossi CE, Wolff WI, Nealon TF et al. (1977) Intraluminal fluorouracil chemotherapy adjunct to surgical procedures for resectable carcinoma of the colon and rectum. Surg Gynecol Obstet 145: 549–554
Hahn RG, Moertel CG, Schutt AJ, Bruckner HW (1975) A double blind comparison of intensive course 5-FU by oral vs intravenous route in the treatment of colorectal carcinoma. Cancer 35: 1031
Hall SW, Tenczynski TF, Benjamin RS, Burgess MA, Valdivieso M, Loo TL, Bodey GP (1978) Clinical, toxicological, and pharmacological studies of combination chemotherapy of adenocarcinoma with adriamycin and Baker's antifolate. Cancer Chemother Pharmacol 1: 139–144
Haller DG, Woolley PV, Macdonald JS, Smith LF, Schein PS (1978) Phase II trial of 5-fluorouracil adriamycin and mitomycin-C in advanced colorectal cancer. Cancer Treat Rep 62: 563
Higgins GA (1976) Chemotherapy, adjuvant to surgery for gastrointestinal cancer. Clin Gastroenterol 5: 795–808
Higgins GA, Dwight RW, Smith JV, Keehn RJ (1971) Fluorouracil as an adjuvant to surgery in carcinoma of the colon. Arch Surg 102: 339–343
Higgins GA, Lee LE, Dwight RW, Keehn RJ (1978) The case for adjuvant 5-fluorouracil in colorectal cancer. Cancer Clin Trials 1: 35–41
Kemeny N, Yagoda A, Burchenal JH (1978) Phase II study of 2,2′-anhydro-1-D-arabinofuranosyl-5-fluorocytosine in advanced colorectal carcinoma. Cancer Treat Rep 62: 463–464
Kisner D, Schein P, Smith L, Cohen P, Smythe TA, Duvall C (1979) 5-Fluorouracil, methyl-CCNU and vincristine (FMV) for colorectal carcinoma: Confirmation of increased response rate using weekly 5-FU. Cancer Treat Rep 63: 982–984
Krause S, Sonoda T, Solomon A (1979) Treatment of advanced-gastrointestinal cancer with 5-fluorouracil and mitomycin C. Cancer 43: 1598–1603
Lawrence W, Terz JJ, Horsley JS, Brown PW, Romero C (1978) Chemotherapy as an adjuvant to surgery for colorectal cancer. Arch Surg 113: 164–168
Livingston RB, Carter SK (1970) Single agents in cancer chemotherapy. IFI/Plenum, New York
Marciniak TA, Moertel CG, Schutt AJ, Hahn RG, Reitemeier RJ (1975) Phase II study of ICRF 159 in advanced colorectal carcinoma. Cancer Chemother Rep 59: 761

Moertel CG (1975) Clinical management of advanced gastrointestinal cancer. Cancer 36: 675–682

Moertel CG (1976) Chemotherapy of gastrointestinal cancer. Clin Gastroenterol 5: 777

Moertel CG (1978) Current concepts in cancer: Chemotherapy of gastrointestinal cancer. N Engl J Med 299: 1049–1052

Moertel CG (1979) Letter. N Engl J Med 301: 329

Moertel CG, Schutt AJ, Hahn RG, Reitemeier RJ (1975) Therapy of advanced colorectal cancer with a combination of 5-fluorouracil, methyl-1,3-cis-(2-chloroethyl)-1-nitrosourea, and vincristine. J Natl Cancer Inst 54: 69

Moertel CG, Schutt AJ, Reitemeier RJ, Hahn RG (1976) Therapy for gastrointestinal cancer with the nitrosoureas alone and in drug combination. Cancer Treat Rep 60: 729

Nair KG, Moayeri H, Mittelman A (1980) A phase II study of fluorodopan in the treatment of advanced colorectal cancer. Cancer Treat Rep 64: 697–699

Oberfield RA, McCaffrey JA, Polio J, Clouse ME, Hamilton T (1979) Prolonged and continuous percutaneous intra-arterial hepatic infusion chemotherapy in advanced metastatic liver adenocarcinoma from colorectal primary. Cancer 44: 414–423

O'Connell MJ, Shani A, Rubin J, Moertel CG (1978) Phase II trial of maytansine in patients with advanced colorectal carcinoma. Cancer Treat Rep 62: 1237–1238

Padilla F, Corres J, Buroker T, Vaitkevicius VK (1978) Phase II study of Baker's antifol in advanced colorectal cancer. Cancer Treat Rep 62: 553–554

Patt YZ, Wallace S, Freireich EJ, Chuang VP, Hersh EM, Mavlight GM (1981) The palliative role of hepatic arterial infusion and arterial occlusion in colorectal carcinoma metastatic to the liver. Lancet 1: 349–351

Rodriguez V, Gottlieb J, Burgess MA et al. (1976) Phase I studies with Baker's antifol (BAF), NSC 139105. Cancer 38: 690–694

Rodriguez V, Richman SP, Benjamin RS et al. (1977) Phase 2 study with Baker's antifol in solid tumors. Cancer Res 37: 980–983

Taylor I, Rowling J, West C (1979) Adjuvant cytotoxic liver perfusion for colorectal cancer. Br J Surg 66: 833–837

Prospects in Management

W. Duncan

Department of Clinical Oncology, University of Edinburgh, Western General Hospital, Edinburgh EH4 2XU, United Kingdom

This presentation is dedicated to the memory of the late George Edelstyn, whom I had the pleasure of knowing during his short professional life. Like all who leave their mark, George Edelstyn was a man of enormous energy and drive. He served on the staff of hospitals in Northern Ireland and in Eire, and his practice took him to many hospitals in both countries. He also found time to be active in local politics, and combining his political and professional talents he was, remarkably, a founder member of three charitable organizations for cancer research. He seemed to have boundless energy, which he directed most successfully in his efforts to improve the care of cancer patients. It is difficult to accept that his untimely death brought to an end so much that was still unfulfilled.

There seems to have been no doubt that radiotherapy and oncology was the speciality for George Edelstyn. Within 3 years of his graduation from Queen's University in Belfast he published his first paper on the *Combination of surgical hypophysectomy and intersellar* ^{90}*Yt irradiation.* There was great debate at that time about the relative merits of radiotherapy, surgery, or a combined approach in effecting the most complete pituitary ablation. I can recall the argument that followed a paper he presented at the Annual General Meeting of this College in Aberdeen. Gordon Stewart had also reported his studies on pituitary ablation by the insertion of ^{90}Yt seeds by the transnasal, transsphenoidal approach. Both were equally committed and vigorous in promoting their different philosophies and practice. Both enjoyed the thrust of debate and both were equally vigorous and articulate in expressing their views. But neither would ever lose the obvious warmth of their personalities. I think all of us who had the privilege of knowing George Edelstyn will always remember his warm and characteristic Irish brogue.

He continued to develop his interests in the management of breast cancer, and became increasingly involved in the use of cytotoxic chemotherapy in the treatment of advanced disease. His major contributions to the literature were in the field of hormonal management and chemotherapy of breast cancer. He was a pathfinder for what was to become the speciality of radiotherapy and oncology. He embraced the concept of total care of the cancer patient and his selfless commitment to his patients and their cause will always be an example for others to follow. It is likely that George Edelstyn would have enjoyed the challenge of improving the management of rectal cancer. It is a disease, like breast cancer, in which the survival rates have shown little change over the last 50 years.

Recent Results in Cancer Research, Vol. 83

Multidisciplinary Approach to Management

The standard surgical procedures for colorectal cancer, such as abdominoperineal excision of the rectum, are largely unchanged and survival rates have not increased in the last 25 years. New techniques in surgery have considerably improved the qualitative results of management and many patients now benefit, in particular, from sphincter-conserving operations. While surgery remains the definitive management for colorectal cancer, there must be more active exploration of the role of adjuvant treatment in the hope of improving survival rates. It is in the development of techniques of combined management that one also may expect to reduce the incidence of loco-regional recurrences and of distant metastases. In the *Compilation of Cancer Therapy Protocol Summaries* (US Department of Health, Education and Welfare 1980), details of 30 clinical trials are given which evaluate adjuvant treatment for apparently localized disease (Table 1). It will be seen that 14 trials are concerned with cytotoxic chemotherapy and 13 with radiotherapy, while 8 trials involve the evaluation of immunotherapy. When one looks at trials of definitive management, other than surgery, it is clear that apart from one exception these new techniques are concerned with the control of metastatic disease (Table 2). In these trials chemotherapy is of principal interest and will be the subject of more detailed discussion later.

Table 1. Collaborative trials in colorectal cancer

Adjuvant treatment	Localized disease	Metastatic disease
Chemotherapy	9	1
Chemotherapy and postop. radiotherapy	4	0
Pre-op. radiotherapy	4	0
Postop. radiotherapy	5	1
Immunotherapy	3	0
Immunotherapy and chemotherapy	5	0
Total	30	2

From *Cancer Therapy Protocols,* US Dept of Health Education and Welfare 1980

Table 2. Collaborative trials in colorectal cancer

Definitive treatment	Localized disease	Metastatic disease
Chemotherapy	0	25
Chemotherapy and Irradiation	1	1
Radiotherapy	0	1
Immunotherapy	0	5
Total	1	32

From *Cancer Therapy Protocols,* US Dept of Health Education and Welfare 1980

Pre-operative Radiotherapy

The most complete series of adjuvant trials has evaluated the role of pre-operative radiotherapy in patients with operable rectal cancer. Five randomly controlled studies have been completed, and three, the Toronto, Memorial, and VASAG I studies, have reported survival data (Table 3). The Veterans Administration Surgical Adjuvant Group (VASAG) has published several reports of its excellently designed and conducted trial of pre-operative radiotherapy (Roswit et al. 1970, 1973). In this study the dose of radiation was 20 gray in ten daily fractions. Some patients with a low-lying cancer were given an additional 5 gray to a perineal field. There was no increase in the operative mortality or morbidity associated with the adjuvant radiotherapy. The first reports (Dwight et al. 1972; Roswit et al. 1975) claimed that there was a significant improvement ($P < 0.05$) in survival for patients who had undergone 'curative' abdominoperineal excision following adjuvant radiotherapy. Longer follow-up has confirmed that survival is better, but not significantly so, for all patients who received pre-operative radiotherapy before abdominoperineal excision (Table 4). The difference in survival remains greatest in patients who had Dukes' C stage cancers. However, the statisticians advise caution in that these differences have been found in subgroups within the main study and consider that a much higher level of statistical significance than 5% should be demanded in these circumstances before it is concluded that the observed differences are real. It is important also to note that there was a significant reduction in the number of patients with Dukes' C cancers in the group given pre-operative radiotherapy, and this fact will be discussed again later. It is of course difficult to explain why patients with Dukes' C rectal cancer, after pre-operative irradiation, should have a better prognosis than the control group. The

Table 3. Pre-operative adjuvant radiotherapy: Completed controlled trials

Group	Radiotherapy	NSD
Toronto	5 gray in 1 fraction	500
Memorial	20 gray in 10 fractions	870
VASAG I	20 gray in 10 fractions	870
MRC I	5 gray in 1 fraction	500
	20 gray in 10 fractions	870
EORTC I	34.5 gray in 15 fractions ± 5 FU	1290

Table 4. Pre-operative radiotherapy in rectal cancer: 5-year survival rates of VASAG I trial

	Irradiated group		Control group	
	No.	Survival	No.	Survival
All patients	347	35.2%	353	28.9%
AP excisions	206	40.8%	208	28.4%
Other resections	96	38.5%	103	39.5%

From Higgins 1978

number of lymph nodes involved has been found to correlate with survival (Copeland et al. 1969) (Table 5). One may suggest that although lymph nodes were found to be involved with tumour histologically, the residual tumour cells were non-viable after irradiation, and these patients might be expected to have a better survival rate than patients with nodes involved with viable cancer. This is a little difficult to accept, as the involvement of regional nodes is an index of the probability of blood-borne metastases. That probability should not be influenced by radiotherapy to the pelvis, although the tumour may be 'down-staged'. Some confirmatory evidence about the benefit of pre-operative radiotherapy is given from the autopsy data obtained from the VASAG trial (Higgins 1978). In an analysis of autopsy data from patients with evidence of rectal cancer at death, it is clear that the number of patients with evidence of cancer at death is significantly reduced in those who received pre-operative irradiation (Table 6). This difference was seen in all patients and not just those who had been managed by abdominoperineal excision.

The Memorial Hospital trial (Stearns et al. 1974) was also a randomly controlled study which compared surgery alone with surgery and adjuvant pre-operative radiotherapy. The dose of radiation, 20 gray in ten daily fractions, was similar to that given in the VASAG I trial. The protocol of this trial has been the subject of criticism, and reservations have been made about the validity of its results. Nonetheless, statistical analysis of survival rates has shown no difference between the irradiated and the control group.

The Toronto trial (Rider et al. 1977) was particularly interesting, as the pre-operative radiotherapy consisted of a single exposure of 5 gray given immediately before, or at most within 8 h, of the operation. A total of 125 patients were included in the trial, and analysis of the actuarial survival rates has shown no difference in the overall results.

Table 5. Rectal cancer: Survival and lymph node involvement

Lymph node involvement	Number of patients	5-Year survival (%)
0	584	51.5
1	112	30.3
2	68	27.9
3	40	17.5
4	24	33.3
>5	110	10.0

From Copeland et al. 1969

Table 6. Pre-operative radiotherapy in rectal cancer: Percentage cancer deaths at autopsy, VASAG I trial

	Irradiated group	Control group
All patients	49%	68%
AP excisions	50%	70%
Other resections	49%	61%
	$P < 0.05$	

From Higgins 1978

However, analysis of the actuarial survival of the small number of patients with Dukes' C cancer, 22 in the irradiated group and 16 in the control group, have demonstrated an improved 5-year survival in the irradiated group, 34% against 18%, which is highly significant ($P = 0.014$). Recently Dr. Rider has confirmed that this difference continues to be observed (1981, personal communication). The 5-year survival rate of 34% for the irradiated group is similar to that reported from the VASAG I trial for patients with Dukes' C cancer (Roswit et al. 1975). The survival of the control group in the Toronto trial is seen to be especially poor.

The EORTC I trial had no control arm of 'surgery alone', and for that reason was discontinued, although the addition of 5-FU was thought to contribute to unacceptably high morbidity. The trial therefore cannot evaluate the benefit of pre-operative radiotherapy, or any increased morbidity with which radiotherapy alone may be associated. The trial compared the effects of a moderate dose of radiotherapy, 34.5 gray given in 15 daily fractions to the whole pelvis (up to the second lumbar vertebra), with or without 5-FU. The 5-FU was given by intravenous infusion in a daily dose of 10 mg/kg for the first 4 days of radiotherapy. It was found that the addition of 5-FU to the radiotherapy significantly increased the serious side-effects. In 121 patients treated with adjuvant radiotherapy alone there were 10 severe complications, compared with 35 observed in 124 patients given radiotherapy and 5-FU (Gerard et al. 1981). These authors found that patients who were especially at risk from combined adjuvant therapy were those over 70 years of age, those with cardiovascular disease, and those with considerable loss of weight. This trial was followed by the EORTC II trial which employs the same regimen of pre-operative radiotherapy (without 5-FU), which is compared with a control group managed by surgery alone. Recruitment to this trial should be completed in mid-1981.

It is also of interest that in many of the trials of pre-operative radiotherapy for rectal cancer there has been a reduction in the proportion of Dukes' C cancers in the irradiated group (Table 7). There are three exceptions. In the trial reported from the Princess Margaret Hospital, Toronto (Rider 1977), there was a smaller percentage (29%) of Dukes' C lesions in the control group than in the group that received 5 gray pre-operatively. The figure of 29% is a little lower than one would expect for the proportion of Dukes' C stage in a large series of rectal cancer patients. Secondly, in the MRC trial, in which 5 gray was given to one group, there was no reduction of Dukes' C cases and the percentage of Dukes' C cases was similar to that in the irradiated group in Toronto. The trial conducted at the Mayo Clinic (Stearns et al. 1974) reported a small but insignificant reduction in Dukes' C cases. The very high

Table 7. Pre-operative radiotherapy in rectal cancer: Proportion of Dukes' C cancers

Group	Irradiated group	Non-irradiated group	Radiotherapy
VASAG I	28%	41%	2 gray × 10
VASAG II	31%	44%	1.75 gray × 18
Mayo	34%	39%	2 gray × 10
Toronto	44%	29%	5 gray × 1
MRC	36%	46%	2 gray × 10
MRC	45%	46%	5 gray × 1
Harvard	29%	69%	1.8 gray × 25

figure (69%) of Dukes' C patients in the control group in the Harvard series (Kligerman 1975, 1977) is exceptional and is much higher than the general experience at Harvard at that time.

The Veterans Administration in 1977 began a second trial of pre-operative radiotherapy (VASAG II), increasing the x-ray dose. In this study 31.5 gray is given in 18 daily fractions, about a 25% increase in dose compared with that employed in the VASAG I trial. It can be seen (Table 7) that there is no difference in the proportion of Dukes' C cancers compared with the first study (Higgins 1979). Survival data have not yet been published for this second trial and they are awaited with great interest.

The Medical Research Council's trial was designed to compare the effects of 20 gray in ten fractions (the VASAG I dose) with 5 gray in one fraction (the Toronto dose). This trial was started in 1975 and closed in 1978, and it is too soon to give an analysis of recurrence or survival rates. Some interesting changes were found after the fractionated course of pre-operative irradiation (MRC Rectal Cancer Working Party, to be published). There was a reduction of the number of Dukes' C cases, as shown in Table 8, the difference from the single fraction and control group just failing to reach the conventional level of statistical significance. There were also significantly fewer patients with cancers under 5.0 cm in diameter in the fractionated treatment group, and compared with the other groups this is a highly significant finding (Table 9). It is evident that the effects of low-dose pre-operative radiotherapy may be observed on the tumour. It is also important to note that in this MRC study there was no increase in postoperative complications following adjuvant radiotherapy. Indeed, there was a significant reduction in anastomotic leaks after both the single- and multiple-fraction radiotherapy. The evidence of significant improvements in survival rates, however, still remains to be obtained.

It may be that higher doses of pre-operative radiotherapy are required before improved survival rates are obtained. A number of other trials are now under way which do use higher doses (Table 10). The VASAG II trial has already been mentioned; the EORTC II trial employs the same dose of pre-operative irradiation as

Table 8. MRC rectal cancer trial: Dukes' stage by treatment allocation

Dukes' stage	No XRT	Single fraction	Ten fractions
A	25.1%	20.8%	22.4%
B	30.3%	33.6%	41.8%
C	44.6%[a]	45.6%	35.9%[a]

[a] $X^2 = 3.53$; $P = 0.06$

Table 9. MRC rectal cancer trial: Tumour size by treatment allocation

Diameter of tumour	No XRT	Single fraction	Ten fractions
1–4	35.8%	41.8%	53.6%
5–7	55.0%	49.2%	40.1%
>8	9.2%	9.0%	6.3%

$X^2 = 15.4$ (4 d.f.); $P = 0.004$

Table 10. Pre-operative adjuvant radiotherapy: Current controlled trials

Group	Radiotherapy	NSD
SWOG	20 gray in 10 fractions ± Mito C and 5-FU	870
VASAG II	31.5 gray in 18 fractions	1110
EORTC II	34.5 gray in 15 fractions	1290
Leningrad/Kiev	30 gray in 6 fractions	1530

used in their first study, but the group receiving 5-FU has been replaced by a 'surgery alone' control arm. The results of this trial are unlikely to be analysed before 1984.

Bruckner et al. (1977) have reported preliminary results of a similar trial in which the same dose of pre-operative radiotherapy (34.5 gray in 15 fractions) was used, showing a reduction in local recurrence. Two other reports, from Leningrad and Kiev, claim improved survival rates after pre-operative radiotherapy (Simbertseva et al. 1975; Zybina and Nabatich 1975). In these trials a relatively high dose of radiation is given, 30 gray in six fractions, with surgery following 2–10 days afterwards. No increase in postoperative complications is associated with this regimen of radiotherapy. Rodriguez-Antunez et al. (1973) have also reported a trial with a similar dose of pre-operative irradiation, 24 gray in three daily fractions, without any additional surgical complications following operation 10–15 days later.

It has also been suggested that radiotherapy may make fixed and inoperable rectal cancers resolve to the extent that they may be successfully excised. Stevens et al. (1976) and Zybina et al. (1977) have given high-dose radiotherapy in the management of these locally advanced lesions and have shown that almost half may become operable. Of course these patients will in all probability have disseminated disease at the time of presentation and it seems doubtful whether adjuvant radiotherapy alone could be expected to improve survival. However, it may be vital part of combined management when effective cytotoxic chemotherapy is found to deal with metastatic disease.

Postoperative Radiotherapy

One important disadvantage and legitimate criticism of pre-operative radiotherapy is that the practice involves treating a proportion of patients who cannot be expected to benefit. About 25% of patients with operable rectal cancer will have an excellent prognosis following surgery alone (Goligher 1981; Nicholls, this volume). The use of pre-operative radiotherapy cannot be justified in these patients. It therefore seems logical to select certain patients, for example those with fixed but operable cancers, for pre-operative radiotherapy. Those with mobile cancers would first have elective surgery, and those found to have more advanced disease or with residual cancer after surgery would proceed to postoperative adjuvant therapy. In the MRC trial it was clearly demonstrated that patients with fixed rectal cancer had a significantly worse prognosis than those with mobile tumours (Fig. 1). In addition, 79% of patients with mobile cancers were considered to have undergone a curative excision, while only 30% of fixed cancers were completely resected. Surgeons were very accurate, as measured

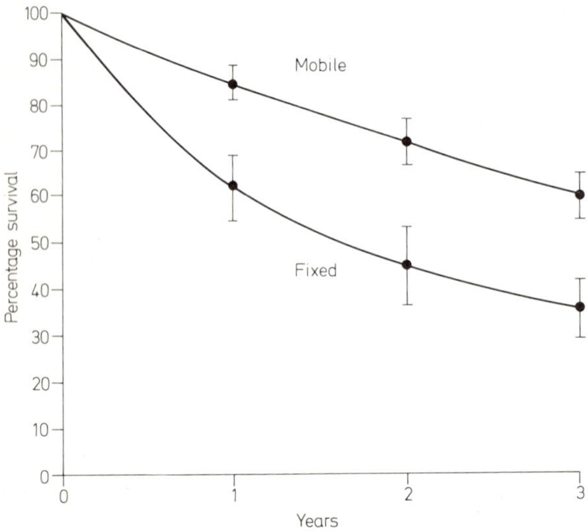

Fig. 1. Actuarial survival rates for patients after resection of mobile or fixed cancer of the rectum

Table 11. Postoperative combined trials after curative resection

Group	Trial
ECOG	RT vs 5-FU + MeCCNU vs RT + CT
GITSG	RT vs 5-FU + MeCCNU vs RT + CT
RTOG	RT vs 5-FU + MeCCNU vs RT + CT

From *Compilation of Cancer Therapy Protocol Summaries* 1980

by survival data, in assessing the completeness of their operation. Patients with fixed rectal cancer determined at the time of pretreatment assessment seem therefore to be a good group on whom to test selectively the effectiveness of pre-operative radiotherapy. Those patients who are found to have mobile tumours are perhaps best managed by primary surgery. Those patients in whom the operation is considered to be incomplete, or who have more advanced lesions, may appropriately be the subject of a trial of postoperative radiotherapy, possibly combined with cytotoxic chemotherapy. More detailed consideration of selection has been reviewed by Gunderson (1976). Three trials of postoperative adjuvant therapy for patients after curative resection are listed in the *Compilation of Cancer Therapy Protocol Summaries* (US Department of Health, Education and Welfare 1980) (Table 11). All have very similar protocols, but the Eastern Cooperative Oncology Group (ECOG) trial does not have a surgery only control arm and so will be of limited value. The Radiation Therapy Oncology Group (RTOG) has closed its protocol without having recruited sufficient patients to the study. The trial conducted by the Gastrointestinal Tumor Study Group (GITSG) in the United States has been most successful, and some exciting interim results have recently been announced. In this GITSG study, patients with Dukes' B2 and C cancer of the rectum who have had a 'curative' abdominoperineal excision are randomly allocated to one of four groups. One group has no further treatment, the second has postoperative radiotherapy, the third postoperative cytotoxic chemotherapy, and the fourth group, both radiotherapy and chemotherapy. The radiotherapy consists of 40–48 gray in 20/28 daily fractions to the pelvis; chemotherapy, in a combination of 5-FU (325 mg/m^2 IV, days 1–5) and methyl-CCNU (130 mg/m^2 by mouth on day 1) given in cycles (every 10 weeks) for 18 months. These doses are modified slightly when both radiotherapy and chemotherapy are given. Further details of the protocol are given in the *Compilation of Cancer Therapy Protocol Summaries* (1980). An interim review (*Clinical Cancer Letter* (1980) has shown that in patients in the group receiving both pre-operative radiotherapy and systemic chemotherapy afterwards there was a significant reduction in the incidence of local recurrence and of distant metastases (Table 12). No improvement in survival rates has yet been observed but the final outcome of this trial cannot be anticipated.

Other groups (Mendiondo et al. 1976; Turner et al. 1977; Friedmann et al. 1978) have also claimed that there is an advantage in postoperative radiotherapy. However, the benefits of postoperative radiotherapy alone require to be confirmed by randomly controlled studies. In the GITSG trial there was no reduction in local recurrence after postoperative radiotherapy alone. A serious concern that is regularly expressed about giving postoperative radiotherapy routinely is the associated rate of morbidity, which may be unacceptably high. Withers and Romsdahl (1977) have reported on 45 patients given radiotherapy after curative resection. It is suggested that the probability is high that this treatment reduced local recurrence but the radiation morbidity was considerable. Four patients had small-bowel obstruction and another had a radionecrosis of the rectum.

Mohiuddin et al. (1980) have sought to obtain the benefits of both pre-operative and postoperative radiotherapy. They have reported the use of a 'sandwich' technique in

Table 12. Rectal cancer: Adjuvant radiotherapy and chemotherapy 2-year results of GITSG trial

Treatment group	Local recurrence	All recurrences
Surgery only	19%	52%
+ Radiotherapy	15%	32%
+ Chemotherapy	23%	39%
+ Radiotherapy/chemotherapy	3%	21%

From Clinical Cancer Letter 1980

Table 13. Postoperative combined trials: Residual, recurrent and unresectable rectal cancer

ECOG I	RT ± 5-FU
ECOG II	RT (+ boost) + 5-FU vs RT (split course) + 5-FU
GITSG	RT (split course) ± 5-FU and MeCCNU ± BCG
Mayo	RT (split course) ± BCG

From *Compilation of Cancer Therapy Protocol Summaries* 1980 which a 5-gray single exposure is given before operation and afterwards a dose of 45 gray in 25 fractions to the pelvis in patients found to have Dukes' stage B_2 and C cancers.

Finally, a number of randomly controlled trials have been started to investigate the role of combined management for patients with residual, recurrent, or non-resectable rectal cancer (Table 13). Outlines of the protocols are given in the *Compilation of Cancer Therapy Protocol Summaries* (1980). These patients have a particularly poor prognosis and one must hope that this multidisciplinary approach may lead to a real improvement in management. Results are not yet available from these studies on patients with locally advanced disease.

Adjuvant Cytotoxic Chemotherapy

A more challenging approach is to search for the combination of cytotoxic agents that will deal effectively with micrometastases. The use of cancerocidal drugs to control subclinical metastatic disease demands that these agents show a high activity and specificity against adenocarcinoma of the gastrointestinal tract. Their toxicity must also be minimal to be acceptable for routine administration to patients who are otherwise fit and well. It is of course essential that the agents are effective in the sites of metastases commonly involved by spread from colonic and rectal cancer. Table 14 shows the relative incidence of the most common sites of metastases from cancer of the colon and rectum. Yagoda and Kameny (1978) have reported their experience of response rates by site of metastases (Table 15). Rather surprisingly, the response rate of metastases in lungs is low compared, for example, with the response of liver or lymph node metastases.

The Eastern Cooperative Oncology Group (ECOG) have reported an excellent evaluation, by randomly controlled trials, of the cytotoxic agents thought to be most active in the treatment of colorectal cancer (Lavin et al. 1980). Their trials included 1,314 patients with advanced colonic or rectal cancer and their assessment was based

Table 14. Metastatic spread by primary site: Percentages with metastases

Primary	Liver	Lung	Peritoneum
Colon	77	30	23
Rectum	63	47	15

$P < 0.001$. From Lavin et al. 1980

Table 15. Chemotherapy of colorectal cancer: Response rates by site

Abdominal recurrence	32%
Liver	24%
Lymph nodes	24%
Subcutaneous tissue	16%
Lungs	8%

After Yagoda and Kameny 1978

on objective tumour response and survival in patients with advanced disease. The drugs, which were given according to carefully designed and monitored protocols, are shown in Tables 16 and 17. No drug or group of drugs tested was better than either oral or intravenous 5-FU (600 mg/m^2 per week). It is disappointing to note that it is now 20 years since 5-FU was introduced for the treatment of gastrointestinal cancer and no more active drug or group of drugs has yet been found.

5-Fluorouracil has been the subject of a number of trials of adjuvant therapy, principally the two published by the Veterans Administration Surgical Adjuvant Group (Higgins et al. 1971, 1976). Both these studies failed to demonstrate any real improvement in survival rates after resection. Grage et al. (1975) also reported a randomly controlled trial of 5-FU given weekly for 12 months postoperatively without any long-term improvement in survival (Moertel 1976). It is therefore with great interest that we await the long-term results of the GITSG trial, which combines postoperative radiotherapy with 5-FU and methyl-CCNU, in view of their remarkable early results.

A technique which is under re-evaluation as showing some promise is hepatic perfusion of cytotoxic drugs. Ansfield et al. (1971) originally attempted to control liver metastases by intra-arterial infusion of 5-FU. Taylor et al. (1979) have suggested that

Table 16. Chemotherapy of colorectal cancer (ECOG studies 1980)

Drug regimen	Patients	Response
5-FU IV	39	15%
5-FU PO	28	18%
5-FU + Cyclo	87	5%
5-FU + 6 T-G	78	10%
MeCCNU	87	15%

Table 17. Chemotherapy of colorectal cancer (ECOG studies 1980)

Drug regimen	Patients	Response
5-FU + MeCCNU	112	9%
5-FU + MeCCNU + VCR	103	11%
5-FU + MeCCNU + DTIC	114	16%
5-FU + hydroxyurea	94	21%

Table 18. Results of hepatic perfusion with 5-FU

	Control group	Treated group
Number of patients	73	66
Liver metastases[a]	13	2
(other metastases)	8	1
Deaths	23	7

[a] $X^2 = 6.7$; $P < 0.01$; From Taylor 1979

perfusion of the portal vein would be more appropriate in management of micrometastases in the liver, since this is their route of spread and their principal blood supply. A randomly controlled study of portal vein infusion with 5-FU and heparin was started in 1975 and interim results have recently been reported (Table 18). Much more detailed assessment of this technique is required, including an examination of the role of heparin itself as an antitumour agent, but the initial experience is most encouraging.

Immunotherapy

Various techniques of immune stimulation are also being developed and investigated, but there is no suggestion at present that they significantly influence the course of the colorectal cancer. The state of the art is well reviewed by Gill (1981) and Mavligit et al. (1978).

Most studies have reported the results of treating patients with advanced disease and have understandably yielded disappointing results. The use of immunotherapy as an adjuvant management for early disease is much more interesting. When there is minimal residual cancer the probability of serological block of a cytotoxic response is smaller and the likelihood of complete tumour regression greater than in patients with advanced disease. Interim reports of randomly controlled trials with *Corynebacterium parvum* (Souter et al. 1979) or modified autologous tumour cells and BCG (B. N. Gray 1981, personal communication) in patients after resection of Dukes' B and C stage cancers have not as yet shown any difference in relapse rates. One other randomly controlled study compares chemotherapy (5-FU and methyl-CCNU) with immunotherapy (MER, a methanol extraction residue of BCG), or a combination of both with surgery alone. It is reported (Lokich 1979) that no difference in relapse or survival rates is evident, but no definite conclusion should be drawn at present. A large number of patients has been recruited for this study, and further analysis after much longer follow-up is awaited with much interest.

Conclusions

An important advance in the last 10 years has been the recognition of the need for a multidisciplinary approach in the management of colorectal cancer. The readiness of increasing numbers of clinicians to collaborate in these demanding studies, particularly in randomly controlled trials, is commendable. However, further encouragement is required to those who find the protocols of trials restrictive of their clinical freedom and prejudicial to their patients' interests. A well-conceived and properly designed trial should not present such difficulties, and in addition clinicians are always free, for any reason, to exclude (before randomization) a particular patient from a controlled trial. But too few patients are included in controlled trials. Tate et al. (1979) have estimated that in the United Kingdom no more than 2% of patients with colorectal cancer are included in comparative studies. In the United Kingdom each year about 23,000 patients present with colorectal cancer, and if only 1 in 10 were to be included in randomly controlled studies our understanding of these diseases and their management would quickly increase.

It is important to pay particular attention to the criteria for the selection of patients for adjuvant treatment. This does require that some simple system of pretreatment assessment be made before a programme of combined management is decided upon. In rectal cancer, mobility has been demonstrated to be of major prognostic significance. In the Medical Research Council's trial of adjuvant radiotherapy for operable rectal cancer 79% of patients with mobile lesions had curative excisions, as opposed to only 30% of patients with fixed cancers. It was also noted that the surgeons' assessment of the completeness of the operation was accurately reflected in the survival rates. Patients with mobile cancers of the rectum have a particularly good prognosis after curative excision. Patients with Dukes' A lesions require no further treatment. Those with Dukes' B and C lesions may benefit by postoperative radiotherapy to the pelvis and systemic cytotoxic chemotherapy. Patients with fixed cancers have a small chance of primary curative excision and accordingly a poor prognosis. Pre-operative radiotherapy may prove to be of selective advantage to this group. Postoperative regional radiotherapy and systemic chemotherapy may also be indicated. This hypothetical outline of a combined approach to management will have to be the subject of a series of controlled trials and there is as yet no good evidence that this policy should be advised in the routine management of patients.

The selection of patients will also depend on accurate pathological staging, tumour grading, and perhaps, in due course, the assay of tumour-specific biochemical markers. Such detailed studies also require data from a large number of patients managed within the protocol of multi-centre trials and carefully followed-up for at least 5 years. It is a demanding challenge to clinical oncologists, but the scientific pursuit of optimum management of potentially curable cancer requires a commitment to a collaborative effort of this magnitude.

It is true that many more patients would be successfully managed today by present surgical techniques alone if the diagnosis could be made at an early stage of tumour development. New methods of early detection are being evaluated (Hardcastle and Vellacott, this volume,) and increasing support must be ensured for this difficult field of laboratory and clinical research. Early diagnosis, although an obvious avenue for clinical progress, is not easy to achieve. However, the introduction of effective population screening leading to earlier diagnosis and timely management could make an impressive contribution to the reduction of mortality rates from colorectal cancer. That must be the major objective until the aetiological factors are accurately defined and their control acceptable socially and politically, so that communities can adopt preventive measures towards eliminating the disease.

References

Ansfield F, Ramirez G, Skibba JL, Bryan GT, Davis HL Jr, Wirtmen GW (1971) Intrahepatic arterial infusion with 5-fluorouracil. Cancer 28: 1147–1158

Bruckner R, Kempf T, Kutzner J, Brunner H (1977) Preliminary results of pre-operative radiotherapy in carcinoma of the rectum. Deutsch Med Wochenschr 102: 195–198

Clinical Cancer Letter (1980) Radio-chemotherapy slashes recurrence rate more than half in GITSG rectal cancer trial. (Editorial) Clinical Cancer Letter 3: 1–3

Copeland EM, Miller LD, Jones RS (1969) Prognostic factors in carcinoma of the colon and rectum. Dis Colon Rectum 10: 415–420

Department of Health, Education and Welfare (1980) Compilation of Cancer Therapy Protocol Summaries, 4th edn. National Institutes of Health, Bethesda (Publication no. 80-1116)

Dwight RW, Higgins GA Jr, Roswit B, LeVeen HH, Keehn RJ (1972) Pre-operative radiation and surgery for cancer of the sigmoid colon and rectum. Am J Surg 123: 93–101

Friedmann P, Park WC, Afonya II, Chabot JR, Garb JL, Pace OT, Emery RW (1978) Adjuvant radiation therapy in colorectal cancer. Am J Surg 135: 512–517

Gerard A, Loygne J, Liegeois A, Kempf P, Camelot G (1981) EORTC clinical trial for treatment of rectal cancer using surgery, radiotherapy and chemotherapy – post operative and delayed complications. In: Gerard A (ed) Progress and perspectives in the treatment of gastrointestinal tumours. Pergamon Press, Oxford, pp 76–82

Gill PG (1981) Immunotherapy. In: DeCosse JJ (ed) Clinical surgery international – Large bowel cancer. Churchill Livingstone, Edinburgh, pp 190–204

Goligher J (1981) Results of operations for large bowel cancer. In: DeCosse JJ (ed) Clinical surgery international – Large bowel cancer. Churchill Livingstone, Edinburgh, pp 154–165

Grage T, Cornell G, Strawitz J, Jones K, Frelick R, Metter G (1975) Adjuvant therapy with 5-FU after surgical resection of colo-rectal cancer. Proc Am Soc Clin Oncol 16: 258–263

Gunderson LL (1976) Radiation therapy: results and future possibilities. Clin Gastroenterol 5: 743–749

Higgins GA Jr (1978) The pros and cons of irradiation treatment in colo-rectal cancer. In: Nyhus LM (ed) Surgery annual. Appleton-Century-Crofts, New York pp 175–190

Higgins GA Jr (1979) Adjuvant radiation therapy in colon cancer. International Advances in Surgical Oncology 2: 1–24

Higgins GA Jr, Dwight RW, Smith JV, Keehn R (1971) Fluorouracil as an adjuvant to surgery in carcinomas of the colon. Arch Surg 102: 339–346

Higgins GA Jr, Humphrey E, Juler CL, LeVeen HH, McCaughan J, Keehn R (1976) Adjuvant chemotherapy in the treatment of large bowel cancer. Cancer 38: 1461–1466

Kligerman MM (1975) Pre-operative radiotherapy in rectal cancer. Cancer 36: 691–695

Kligerman MM (1977) Radiotherapy and rectal cancer. Cancer 39: 896–900

Lavin P, Mittelman A, Douglass H Jr, Engstrom P, Klaassen D (1980) Survival and response to chemotherapy for advanced colorectal adenocarcinoma. An Eastern Cooperative Oncology Group Report. Cancer 46: 1536–1543

Lokich JJ (1979) Adjuvant therapy for surgically curable colon cancer: a controlled study of chemo and immune therapy. Proc Am Soc Cancer Res 20: 423–428

Mavligit GM, Gutterman JU, Hersh EM (1978) Adjuvant chemotherapy and immunotherapy in colorectal cancer. In: Lipkin M, Good RA (eds) Gastrointestinal tract cancer. Plenum Medical, New York, pp 573–589

Medical Research Council Rectal Cancer Working Party (to be published) A trial of pre-operative radiotherapy in the management of operable rectal cancer. First Report Lancet

Mendiondo OA, Wang CC, Welch JP, Donaldson GA (1976) Postoperative radiotherapy in carcinoma of the rectum and distal sigmoid colon. Radiology 119: 673–676

Moertel CG (1976) Fluorouracil as an adjuvant to colorectal cancer surgery: The breakthrough that never was. JAMA 236: 1935–1948

Mohiuddin M, Dobelbower RR, Kramer S (1980) A new approach to adjuvant radiotherapy in rectal cancer. Int J Radiat Oncol Biol Phys 6: 205–207

Rider WD, Palmer JA, Mahoney LJ, Robertson CT (1977) Pre-operative irradiation in operable cancer of the rectum: report of the Toronto trial. Can J Surg 20: 335–338

Rodriguez-Antunez A, Chernak ES, Jelden GL, Hunter TW (1973) Pre-operative irradiation of carcinoma of the rectum. Radiology 108: 689–690

Roswit B, Higgins GA Jr, Keehn RJ (1970) A controlled study of pre-operative irradiation in cancer of the sigmoid colon and rectum. Radiology 97: 133–140

Roswit B, Higgins GA Jr, Humphrey EW, Robinette CD (1973) Pre-operative irradiation of operable adenocarcinoma of the rectum and recto-sigmoid. Radiology 108: 389–395

Roswit B, Higgins GA Jr, Keehn RJ (1975) Pre-operative irradiation for carcinoma of rectum and recto-sigmoid colon – Report of National Veterans Administration randomized study. Cancer 35: 1597–1602

Simbirtseva LP, Sneshko LI, Smirov NM (1975) Results of intensive combined therapy for carcinoma of the rectum. Vopr Onkol 21: 7–12

Souter R, Gill PG, Morris PJ (1979) Trial of adjuvant immunotherapy with *Corynebacterium parvum*. Cited in Gill (1981)

Stearns MW Jr, Deddish MR, Quan SHQ, Leaming RH (1974) Pre-operative roentgen therapy for cancer of the rectum and recto-sigmoid. Surg Gynaecol Obstet 138: 584–586

Stevens KR Jr, Allen CV, Fletcher WS (1976) Pre-operative radiotherapy for carcinoma of the rectosigmoid. Cancer 37: 2866–2874

Tate H, Rawlinson J, Freedman LS (1979) How many British cancer patients are enrolled in comparative treatment studies? Lancet 2: 623–625

Taylor I, Rowling JT, West C (1979) Adjuvant liver perfusion for colorectal cancer. Br J Surg 66: 833–837

Turner SS, Vieira EF, Ager PJ, Alpert S, Efron G, Ragins H, Weil P, Ghossein NA (1977) Elective postoperative radiotherapy for locally advanced colorectal cancer. A preliminary report. Cancer 40: 105–108

Wassif SB (1974) A pilot study of a new regime of combined therapy for the radical treatment of marginally operable rectal (or colorectal) cancer. Eur J Cancer 10: 615–619

Withers HR, Romsdahl MM (1977) Postoperative radiotherapy for adenocarcinoma of the rectum and rectosigmoid. Int J Radiat Oncol Biol Phys 2: 1069–1071

Yagoda A, Kameny N (1978) Chemotherapy of colorectal cancer: A critical analysis of response criteria and therapeutic efficacy. In: Lipkin M, Good RA (eds) Gastrointestinal cancer. Plenum Medical, New York, pp 551–572

Zybina MA, Nabatich NN (1975) Results of combination treatment for rectal cancer. Vestn Khir 114: 67–69

Zybina MA, Chernichenko VA, Lute-Pokrovskaia TA, Arungazyera VV, Zaichuk AI (1977) Combined treatment of immobile rectal cancer with the use of preoperative intensive fractionated irradiation. Khirugiia (Mosk) 10: 72–76

Subject Index

abdomino-perineal excision 106
abdomino-sacral operations 106
abscess pelvic 106
acute phase reactant proteins 72
adenocarcinoma 50
adenoma 50, 77, 87
–, barium-enema 77
–, histology 48, 59
–, hyperplastic 53
–, incidence 45
– tubular 50, 59
–, tubulo-villous 50
–, villous 50, 59
adenoma-carcinoma sequence 45, 47, 50, 87
adjuvant management 136
– –, chemotherapy 131
– –, immunotherapy 146
– –, radiotherapy 136
adriamycin 127
Adventists californian 12
Africa 15
age incidence 87
albumin 67, 74
α, anti-trypsin 73
amoebiasis 37
anaplastic carcinoma 106
–, restorative operation 106
anastomosis, hand-sutured 107
–, leakage 106
–, stapled 106
anterior resection 106
antibodies 41
anti-CEA antibodies 95
– –, radio-labelled scanning 95
anti-chymotrypsin 73
antigen-antibody 39
antigen, carcino-embryonic 38, 67
–, lymphocyte 39
antimetabolites 127
anti-sera, human haemaglobin 92
–, immunofluorescence 94
–, radial immunodiffusion 92
arterial infusion chemotherapy 130
autologous tumour cells 146
azathioprine 34

B-lymphocytes 40
bacterial flora 12
Baker's antifol 127
barium enema 24, 77
– –, double contrast 24
– –, examples 33, 37
– –, vs colonscopy 84
– suspension 79
BCG 146
beer 13,17
benzidine test 89
benzopyrene hydroxylase 16
Beta-carotene 25
bile salts 12
biochemical markers 67
bladder dysfunction 104
bleeding, occult faecal 89
–, recurrent disease 113
Bombay 13
Brazil 1
Brewery workers 17
buscopan 80

C-reactive protein 67, 73
Canada 1, 12
cancer families 53
carcino-embryonic antigen 38, 67
– – in faeces 94
– –, selection for treatment 117
– – in serum 95
– –, survival rates 69, 118
carcinogenesis 28
caucasians 2
cell cycle phases 22
– – time 22

– loss factor 23, 26
– population kinetics 21
– – – colorectal cancer 27
– – – normal mucosa 27
– production 21
– – rates 26
– – normal mucosa 26
– – rectal cancer 26
cellular heterogeneity 28
chemotherapy 126
– adjuvant 131
–, arterial infusion 130
–, monitoring progress 71
–, umbilical vein 132, 145
Chinese 1, 12
chromagenic indicators 89
chromium, radioactive labelling 89
cleansing enema 78
clinical trials, collaborative 136
– –, chemotherapy 126
– –, immunotherapy 146
– –, radiotherapy 137
clonogenicity 128
clonogenic cells 29
coeliac disease 36
colitis amoebic 37
– ischaemic 38
–, radiation induced 36
–, schistosomiasis 37
–, tuberculous 38
colonal anastomosis 107
colonic lavage 94
colonoscopy, compared barium enema 84
–, tumour detection 87
colorectal anastomosis 108
combination chemotherapy 128
combined management, see multidisciplinary management
compliance rates screening 92
computerized tomography 77
contact radiotherapy 108, 119
controlled trails, see clinical trials
Copenhagen 14
corticosteroids 34
corynebacterium parvum 146
Crohn's disease 34
crypt cells 21
cyclophosphamide 129
cytotoxic chemotherapy 126, 144
Czechoslovakia 31

dairy products 13
Denmark 1, 18, 31
diagnosis, early 86
dietary factors 11
– fibre 16
differentiation, cell 22
–, tumour 59
discharge 113
diverticular disease 38
DNA synthesis 22
double contrast enema 78
– – –, barium suspension 79
– – –, contra-indications 77
– – –, growth measurements 24
– – –, preparation 78
– – –, radiographs 33, 37, 81
– – –, technique 80
doubling time 24
DTIC 145
Dukes' stage
– –, carcino-embryonic antigen 68
– –, distribution general 101
– –, – polyposis coli 52
– –, extra mural infiltration 61
– –, survival rates 60, 69, 77, 86
– –, tumour markers 68
– –, venous invasion 64
dysplasia 32, 48, 59, 84
–, radiological appearances 84

electrofulgurisation 108
endocavitary irradiation 119
England and Wales 1, 13
environmental factors 45, 56
epithelial dysplasia 32, 48, 59, 84
ethnic differences in cancer risk 31
extra-mural infiltration 61, 65, 109
– –, Dukes' stage 61

faecal fistula 106
– occult blood 89
– – –, criteria for tests 89
FAM regimen 130
familial cancers 53
– polyposis coli 45, 84, 87
fat intake 12
fats 14
fecatest 90
fibre, dietary 13
–, –, pentose fraction 16
Finland 1, 12, 14
fish 13
fistula, faecal 106
flow cytometry 28
5-fluorocytosine 128
5-fluorodeoxyuridine 131

fluorodopan 127
5-fluorouracil 113, 127, 143, 145
– and Xray therapy 114, 120, 139
fraction labelled mitosis 25
fruit 13
– vegetables 14
Ftorafur 127

gamma-glutamyl transpeptidase 67
genetic factors 11, 45
geographical variations 1, 31
glucagon 80
gluten enteropathy 36
glycoprotein 73
growth curve 24
– fraction 22
Guaiac test 89

haemaglobin level in stool 89
haematin component 89
haemoccult test 89
– – false-negative rate 91
haptoglobin 73
Hawaii 13
hematest 90
heparin 146
hepatic metastases 63
– –, arterial infusion 130
– –, venous infusion 132, 145
– resection 109
heterogeneity, see cellular heterogeneity
high anterior resection 107
– arterial ligation 103
histiocytosis, malignant 36
Hungary 1, 12
hydroxyurea 145
hyoscine butylbromide 79
hyperbaric oxygen 121
– –, irradiation 121
hyperplasia adenoma 53
– reactive 33
hyperplastic polyps 87
hypersensitivity reactions 40

Iceland 1, 12
immune complex hypersensitivity 41
immuno-chemical tests 67, 92
immuno-deficiency disease 38
immunodiffusion techniques 92
immunofluorescent techniques 94
immunological methods, hemaglobin detection 92
– reactions 31, 39
immunotherapy 146
indicence rates 1 ff.
indoles 16
inflammation 31
– and colon cancer
inheritance, polyposis coli 53
inoperable rectal cancer, chemotherapy 128
– – – immunotherapy 146
– – – radiotherapy 114
intra-arterial chemotherapy 130
Israel 1, 12, 13, 31

Jamaica 1, 12
Japan 1, 12
Japanese in USA 12

kinetics, cell 21
Kuopia 14

labelled mitosis 25
labelling index 23
lager 18
laser destruction 108
latent period 59
leiomyosarcoma 50
liquid paraffin 18
liver metastases, see hepatic metastases
Liverpool 17
liver scan 117
local excision, criteria for 108
– recurrence 63, 124
– –, CEA levels 110
– –, elective surgery 109
– –, radiotherapy 114
– – rates 109, 123, 143
– – – after adjuvant therapy 143
– – –, coloanal anastomosis 107
– –, –, second look' surgery 110
low anterior resection 107
– arterial ligation 103
lung metastases 63
– –, growth measurement 25
lymph node metastases 61, 104, 108
– – –, pre-operative irradiation 139
– – –, survival 138
lymphadenectomy extended 104
– pelvic 104
lymphocytes intra-epithelial 39
–, lamina propria 39
–, subclasses 40
lymphoma 33, 36, 38, 50

macroscopic appearances 62
main vessel ligation 103
Malmö method 80
Malta 1
maytansine 128
meat consumption 12, 14
Medical Research Council, register coeliac disease 36
megavoltage irradiation 113
melphalan 127
Memorial Sloan Kettering Cancer Center 86
MER 146
mesenteric clearance 103
mesothelioma 11
metaphase arrest 26
metastases, chemotherapy 128, 144
–, distribution 63, 144
–, incidences 63
–, – after combined therapy 143
–, – – radiotherapy 138
–, markers 71
–, surgical management 109
methotrexate 127
methyl-CCNU 127, 143, 145
metronidazole 128
microadenoma 52
milk 13
Minnesota Cancer Detection Center 86
mitomycin-C 127
monitoring progress, biochemical markers 70, 146
– –, CEA 70, 110
– –, chemotherapy 71
monoclonal CEA assay 72
morbidity, chemotherapy 128
– combined treatments 116
– radiotherapy 116
– surgery 107
Mormons 14
morphology, tumour 62
mortability rates 7, 86
– – operative 104
mucoid carcinoma 31, 36
mucosa, normal 21
multidisciplinary management 136
– –, chemotherapy 113
– –, post-operative irradiation 142, 121
– –, pre-operative irradiation 122, 137
multivariate analysis 68

Negroes 2
neurogenic bladder 104
neutron irradiation 120
New Zealand 1, 12
Nigeria 1, 12
nitrosourea 127
Norway 1, 12, 13
no touch technique 104
Nuns 14

obstruction, survival 86
occult blood, see faecal occult blood
operative mortality 102, 104
– –, abdomino-perineal excision 104
– –, abdomino-sacral procedures 108
– –, anterior resection 106
– –, causes 106
– –, colo-anal anastomosis 107
– –, pull-through procedures 108
orosomucoid 73
orthotolidine 89

pain, radiotherapy for 113
palliative treatment 113
pathology 59
pelvic lymphadenectomy 104
peranal anastomosis 106
peroheme-40 test 90
peroxidase test 89
phaechromocytoma 80
phases, cell cycle 22
plasma proteins 72
polypectomy 57
polypoid lesions, radiology 81
polyposis coli 11, 45
– –, indicence 57
– –, inheritance 53
– –, St. Marks' Hospital Register 59
– –, surgery 46
polyps hyperplastic 87
perforation, survival 86
Poland 1, 12
post-operative mortality, see operative mortality
– radiotherapy 124, 141
– –, morbidity 143
potential doubling time 22
pre-albumin 67
premalignant changes 87
pre-operative radiotherapy 122, 137, 140
prevention 56
proctosigmoidoscopy for screening 88
prognostic factors 68, 101
– –, arterial ligation 104
– –, Dukes' stage 102
– –, extramural invasion 102
– –, histological grade 102

– –, resectability rate 103
– –, surgery 103
– –, ulcerative colitis 31
proliferation index 22
– unit 21
pro-vitamin A 15
pull-through procedures 106
pulse labelling 25
pyrazofurin 128

radiation-induced colitis 36
radical operations, survival 102
radiological appearances, colon cancer
radiology 77
radionuclide imaging 77
– implantation 119
radioresistance 113
radiosensitizers 120
radiotherapy 113
– adjuvant 122, 137
– contact 108
– definitive 116
– interstitial 119
–, megavoltage 113
–, neutron 120
–, orthovoltage 113
– palliative 115
– post-operative 124, 141
– pre-operative 122, 137
–, split-course 120
razoxone 128
reactions, antigen-antibodies 39
–, antigen-lymphocyte 39
–, hypersensitivity 40
reaginic hypersensitivity 41
recurrence rates 63
– –, see local recurrence rates
– –, see metastases rates
recurrent disease 63
– –, markers 71
red cell radioactive labelling 89
religious orders 14
resectability rate 103
response rates, chemotherapy 127
– –, metastases 144
– –, radiotherapy 116
restorative operations 106
– –, abdominosacral operation 106
– –, anterior resection 106
– –, coloanal anastomosis 107
– –, colorectal anastomosis 108
– –, peranal anastomosis 106
– –, pull-through procedures 108
– resection 105, 106
retinol-binding protein 73
retrorectal lymph notes 108
rubidazone 128

salazopyrin 34
schistosomiasis 37
scopolamine 79
Scotland 1, 12
screening, population 57, 88
–, – compliance rates 92
–, – haemoccult test 93
second-look operations 110
sialomucins 95
sigmoidoscopy 88
Singapore 1
size tumour 62
– –, pre-operative XRT 140
small bowel cancer 34
Spain 1
sphincter-conserving operations 105
split-course radiotherapy 120
St. Marks' Hospital 59, 101
– –, polyposis register 46
– –, surgical results 60
stapling devices 106
stathmokinetic techniques 26
stem cells 21
stenosis annular 81
– segmental 81
stout 17
surgery 101
–, factors in prognosis 103
– for polyposis coli 46
survival rates 9
– –, abdomino-perineal excision 101
– –, abdomino-sacral procedures 108
– –, anterior resection 106
– –, coloanal anastomosis 107
– –, Dukes' stage 6, 77, 86, 126, 138
– –, extra mural invasion 61
– –, fixed cancers 119, 142
– –, histology 102
– –, inoperable cancers 116, 117
– –, liver resection 109
– –, lymph node involvement 86, 138
– –, mobile cancers 119
– –, radiotherapy 119, 124, 137, 142
– –, sphincter-conserving operations 107
– –, surgery 101
– –, tumour morphology 62
– –, – size 62
survivorship function 75
Sweden 1, 12

Switzerland 1, 12
synchronous cancers 51

T-cell 39
– mediated immune reactions 40, 42
tenesmus 113
6-thioguanine 129
transferrin 67
triazinate 127
tritiated thymidine 23
tuberculosis 38
tubular adenoma 50
– – malignancy 87
tubulo-villous adenoma 87
tumour associated antigens in faeces 94
tumour localization, radiolabelled antibodies 95
tumour diameter 62
– markers 67
– – pre, post operative 68
– morphology 62
– –, survival 63
– –, venous infiltration 64
Turnbull excision 104

ulcerative colitis 31, 59
– –, cancer risk 32, 38
ultrasonography 77, 117
USA 1, 12, 17

vegetables 13, 14
venous invasion 63, 109
– –, tumour morphology 64
villous adenoma 5, 87, 801
– –, malignancy 87
– –, radiology 81
vincristine 26, 129
vitamin A 13, 15

Wales 1, 13

X-irradiation 116
–, see radiotherapy

Yorkshire GI Cancer Research Group 67
Yugoslavia 1

Zimbabwe 1

Recent Results in Cancer Research

Sponsored by the Swiss League against Cancer. Editor in Chief: P. Rentchnick, Genève

For information about Vols. 1–9, please contact your bookseller of Springer-Verlag

10 NELSON, R. S.: Radioactive Phosphorus in the Diagnosis of Gastrointestinal Cancer.
11 FREEMAN, R. G. and J. M. KNOX: Treatment of Skin Cancer.
12 LYNCH, H. T.: Hereditary Factors in Carcinoma.
13 Tumours in Children, 2nd Edition. Edited by H. B. MARSDEN and J. K. STEWARD.
14 ODARTCHENKO, N.: Production Cellulaire Erythropoïétique.
15 SOKOLOFF, B.: Carcinoid and Serotonin.
16 JACOBS, M. L.: Malignant Lymphomas and Their Management.
17 Normal and Malignant Cell Growth. Edited by R. J. M. FRY, M. L. GRIEM, and W. H. KIRSTEN (Symposium).
18 ANGLESIO, E.: The Treatment of Hodgkin's Disease.
19 BANNASCH, P.: The Cytoplasm of Hepatocytes during Carcinogenesis. Electron- and Lightmicroscopical Investigations of the Nitrosomorpholineintoxicated Rat Liver.
20 Rubidomycin. A new Agent against Cancer. Edited by J. BERNARD, R. PAUL, M. BOIRON, C. JACQUILLAT, and R. MARAL.
21 Scientific Basis of Cancer Chemotherapy. Edited by G. MATHÉ (Symposium).
22 KOLDOVSKÝ, P.: Tumor Specific Transplantation Antigen.
23 FUCHS, W. A., J. W. DAVIDSON, and H. W. FISCHER: Lymphography in Cancer. With contributions by G. JANTET AND H. RÖSLER.
24 HAYWARD, J.: Hormones und Human Breast Cancer. An Account of 15 Years Study.
25 ROY-BURMAN, P.: Analogues of Nucleic Acid Components. Mechanisms of Action.
26 Tumors of the Liver. Edited by G. T. PACK and A. H. ISLAMI.
27 SZYMENDERA, J.: Bone Mineral Metabolism in Cancer.
28 MEEK, E. S.: Antitumour and Antiviral Substances of Natural Origin.
29 Aseptic Environments and Cancer Treatment. Edited by G. MATHÉ (Symposium).
30 Advances in the Treatment of Acute (Blastic) Leukemias. Edited by G. MATHÉ (Symposium).
31 DENOIX, P.: Treatment of Malignant Breast Tumors. Indications and Results.
32 NELSON, R. S.: Endoscopy in Gastric Cancer.
33 Experimental and Clinical Effects of L-Asparaginase. Edited by E. GRUNDMANN and H. F. OETTGEN (Symposium).
34 Chemistry and Biological Actions of 4-Nitroquinolin 1-Oxide. Edited by H. ENDO, T. ONO, and T. SUGIMURA.
35 PENN, I.: Malignant Tumors in Organ Transplant Recipients.
36 Current Concepts in the Management of Lymphoma and Leukemia. Edited by J. E. ULTMANN, M. L. GRIEM, W. H. KIRSTEN, and R. W. WISSLER (Symposium).
37 CHIAPPA, S., R. MUSUMECI, and C. USLENGHI: Endolymphatic Radiotherapy in Malignant Lymphomas. With contributions by G. BONADONNA, B. DAMASCELLI, G. FAVA, F. PIZZETTI, U. VERONESI.
38 KOLLER, P. C.: The Role of Chromosomes in Cancer Biology.
39 Current Problems in the Epidemiology of Cancer and Lymphomas. Edited by E. GRUNDMANN and H. TULINIUS (Symposium).
40 LANGLEY, F. A. and A. C. CROMPTON: Epithelial Abnormalities of the Cervix Uteri.
41 Tumours in a Tropical Country. A Survey of Uganda (1964–1968). Edited by A. C. TEMPLETON.
42 Breast Cancer: A Challenging Problem. Edited by M. L. GRIEM, E. V. JENSEN, J. E. ULTMANN, and R. W. WISSLER (Symposium).
43 Nomenclature, Methodology and Results of Clinical Trials in Acute Leukemias. Edited by G. MATHÉ, P. POUILLART, L. SCHWARZENBERG (Symposium).
44 Special Topics in Carcinogenesis. Edited by E. GRUNDMANN (Symposium).
45 KOLDOVSKÝ, P.: Carcinoembryonic Antigens.
46 Diagnosis and Therapy of Malignant Lymphoma. Edited by K. MUSSHOFF (Symposium).
47 Investigation and Stimulation of Immunity in Cancer Patients. Edited by G. MATHÉ and R. WEINER (Symposium).
48 Platinum Coordination Complexes in Cancer Chemotherapy. Edited by T. A. CONNORS and J. J. ROBERTS (Symposium).
49 Complications of Cancer Chemotherapy. Edited by G. MATHÉ and R. K. OLDHAM (Symposium).
50 Cancer Registry, Edited by E. GRUNDMANN and E. PEDERSEN (Symposium).
51 Gliomas. Current Concepts in Biology, Diagnosis and Therapy. Edited by J. HEKMATPANAH (Symposium).

52 The Ambivalence of Cytostatic Therapy. Edited by E. GRUNDMANN and R. GROSS (Symposium).
53 A. CLARYSSE, Y. KENIS, and G. MATHÉ: Cancer Chemotherapy.
54 Malignant Bone Tumors. Edited by E. GRUNDMANN.
55 MATHÉ, G.: Cancer Active Immunotherapy, Immunoprophylaxis, and Immunorestoration.
56 Lymphocytes, Macrophages, and Cancer. Edited by G. MATHÉ, I. FLORENTIN, and M.-C. SIMMLER (Symposium).
57 Breast Cancer: A Multidisciplinary Approach. Edited by G. ST. ARNEAULT, P. BAND, and L. ISRAËL (Symposium).
58 B. S. SCHOENBERG: Multiple Primary Malignant Neoplasms.
59 Selective Heat Sensitivity of Cancer Cells. Edited by A. ROSSI-FANELLI, R. CAVALIERE, B. MONDOVI, and G. MORICCA.
60 Tumors of the Male Genital System. Edited by E. GRUNDMANN and W. VAHLENSIECK (Symposium).
61 D. METCALF: Hemopoietic Colonies.
62 Tactics and Strategy in Cancer Treatment. Edited by G. MATHÉ (Symposium).
63 Antitumor Antibiotics. Edited by S. K. CARTER, H. UMEZAWA, J. DOUROS, and Y. SAKURAI (Symposium).
64 Lymphoid Neoplasias I: Classification, Categorization, Natural History.
65 Lymphoid Neoplasias II: Clinical and Therapeutic Aspects.
Lymphoid Neoplasias I & II. Proceedings of the 1977 CNRS-EORTC International Colloquium. Editors: G. MATHÉ, M. SELIGMANN, M. TUBIANA. Devided into two volumes.
66 Carcinogenic Hormones. Edited by C. H. LINGEMAN.
67/68 Adjuvant Therapies and Markers of Post-Surgical Minimal Residual Disease I & II. Proceedings of the 1978 Annual Plenary Meeting of the EORTC. Editors: G. BONADONNA, G. MATHÉ, S. E. SALMON. Divided into two volumes.
67 Markers and General Problems of Cancer Adjuvant Therapies.
68 Adjuvant Therapies of the Various Primary Tumors.
69 Strategies in Clinical Hematology. Edited by R. GROSS and K.-P. HELLRIEGEL.
70 New Anticancer Drugs. Edited by S. K. CARTER
71 Endocrine Treatment of Breast Cancer. Edited by B. HENNINGSEN, F. LINDER, C. STREICHELE.
72 CAWLEY, J. C., BURNS, G. F., HAYHOE, F. G. J.: Hairy-Cell Leukaemia.
73 Thyroid Cancer. Edited by W. DUNCAN.
74 Cancer Chemo- and Immunopharmacology. 1. Chemopharmacology. Edited by G. MATHÉ and F. M. MUGGIA.
75 Cancer Chemo- and Immunopharmacology. 2. Immunopharmacology, Relations and General Problems. Edited by G. MATHÉ and F. M. MUGGIA.
76 New Drugs in Cancer Chemotherapy. Edited by S. K. CARTER, Y. SAKURAI, H. UMEZAWA
77 K. STANLEY, J. STJERNSWÄRD, M. ISLEY: The Conduct of a Cooperative Clinical Trial.
78 Prostate Cancer. Edited by W. DUNCAN.
79 Chemotherapy and Radiotherapy of Gastrointestinal Tumors. Edited by H. O. KLEIN.
80 Adjuvant Therapies of Cancer. Edited by G. MATHÉ, G. BONADONNA, S. SALMON.
81 H. P. LOHRMANN and W. SCHREML: Cytotoxic Drugs and the Granulopoietic System.
82 Early Detection and Localization of Lung Tumors in High Risk Groups. Edited by P. R. BAND.
83 Colorectal Cancer. Edited by W. DUNCAN.